# WORKING
## WITH YOUR
# CHAKRAS

# WORKING
## WITH YOUR
# CHAKRAS

## RUTH WHITE

PIATKUS

First published in 1993 by
Judy Piatkus (Publishers) Ltd of
5 Windmill Street, London W1T 2JA

Reprinted 1994, 1995, 1996, 1997, 1998 (three times), 1999, 2000

**The moral right of the author
has been asserted**

*A catalogue record for this book is
available from the British Library*
ISBN 0–7499–1264–2

Designed by Sue Ryall
Illustrations by Hugh Dunsford-Wood

Set in Compugraphic Baskerville by
Action Typesetting Ltd, Gloucester
Printed and bound in Great Britain by Biddles Ltd
*www.biddles.co.uk*.

To Grace Goodman, for her wise compassion, her delight in life, her generosity and unfailing encouragement.

# Acknowledgements

Many friends, through practical support, words of encouragement, and raising of spirits, have helped me in the writing of this book. I thank them all for 'being there' and for 'seeing me through'.

Particular tributes go to Lorna St Aubyn for unfailing help and encouragement of all kinds; to Professor Eric Gomes for fruitful discussions; to my daughter Jane for much down to earth assistance; to Hugh Dunsford-Wood for the diagram on page 5; and above all, to Tony Van den Bergh for correcting the final script with love, humour and precision.

# Contents

# Foreword

Our society has lost touch with the principles of measurement, harmony and unity known and expressed by many ancient cultures. Although interest in, and use of, these Divine proportions had a revival during the Renaissance period, in our present relationship with nature it is clear that any sense of rapport or synthesis has almost completely disappeared.

In a changing way of thinking, we are, once again, in search of spiritual and eternal values. This is certainly one of the main reasons for the great interest in the chakra system and for the multitude of books and drawings published, and workshops organized, on the subject today.

What is this chakra system? Most of the classical esoteric books describe it as an ancient Indian way of dealing with the energy currents of the human body.

It is not so commonly known that this system was recognized in the West and used in calculating the measurements and proportions of some of our great Cathedrals.

Ancient Indian yoga, one of six orthodox darshanas, 'ways' or philosophies, describes the main structure of the human energy body as six centres or chakras. These also refer to different levels of consciousness, and are often represented as padmas or lotus flowers. A seventh chakra above the head is also included, but in Indian tradition, this one does not belong directly to the human body.

Apart from these six-plus-one main chakras or padmas, there are many other whirlpools of energy essential to the forming and building up of the physical body – in the shoulders, the elbows, the wrists, the hips, knees and ankles. My personal work has made me aware of even more energy centres in the body than those usually described. Every spinal vertebra, for instance, is alive with subtle movement – the Latin 'vertere' means 'to turn'.

The whole chakra system could be compared with a magnetic field from which iron filings will take a pattern – thus the human physical body gets its structure from its energy field.

In the Indian chakra system one character of the Devanagari or Sanskrit alphabet is written on each petal of the first six chakras. The rhythms built up by these characters in the chakras correspond with the number of vertebrae in the spine and with other important anatomical details.

The seventeenth-century German author, J. G. Gichtel, in his book *Theosophica Practica*, places the planets in relationship to the human body, in a similar way to the chakras. Thus the Moon becomes the first chakra, Mercury the second, Venus the third, the Sun the fourth, Mars the fifth, Jupiter the sixth and Saturn the seventh. (In ascending order.)

Drawings showing the complete movement of these planets not only confirm the numbers of petals of every chakra and the anatomical patterns, but also reflect the way in which the Sanskrit characters are written on the lotus flowers. One character out of place would disturb the whole system.

The chakra system expresses the unity of the universe, the unity of the human being and the underlying harmony of both. Of this there is confirmation in the fundamental

Hermetic (and Tantric) wisdom: 'as above, so below', and 'every human being is an indivisible part of the Universe and is, in itself, an expression of that Universe'.

Working with the chakra system will enable us to experience our inner unity and harmony, which in its turn, will lead us to renew our knowledge of the unity and harmony of the Universe.

The question remains, 'How are we, as Westerners to become conscious of this magnificent instrument of inner and outer experience and to proceed in learning to work with it?' There are various ways to do so – such as through different kinds of yoga, all of which demand competent teaching, combined with the patience to train body and mind. There are also techniques which come more directly from our own culture.

This book outlines a mainly Western approach. The information given will enable the reader to have direct experience of the chakras and of the energy flow in the body. With the aid of psychology, esoteric teachings, crystals, colours, fragrances, meditations and visualizations, Ruth White leads the reader, step-by-step, into a new and refreshing world. Her knowledge comes from many years of running workshops on the subject, information from Gildas (her discarnate guide), and from the personal path of growth she has had the strength and courage to undertake.

It will be apparent to the attentive reader that colours and other details do not always conform to the ancient Indian symbolism, or to what other authors have written. This could, though should not, lead to confusion. We are used to the Western scientific logic where there is severe categorization. *Tertium non datur* – a third vision is excluded. This way of thinking has, in the past, been useful to some extent, but modern scientific paradigms are changing to include the position from which several points of view can be true at the same time.

An old Indian priest told me how to see these paradoxes: 'Suppose that between you and me there are three towers.

Two of the towers are standing on one axis. The third one is standing out of the axis. Now, I ask you, "Where does the third tower stand? On your right or left side?" You will say, for instance: "On the right side", but for me that will be on the left (or vice versa)'.

This book is written to give you, the reader, the opportunity of exploring your own energy field and consciousness. Sooner or later you will find out what is true for yourself at any given moment. If you have understood an implicit message of the book you will know also that another's different experience can be true at the same time. At that moment the world will have become a little more harmonious and a little more one.

*Professor Eric Gomes*
*Ghent, Belgium, 1993*

# Chapter 1

# Exploring
# Your Chakras

'Gildas', my discarnate guide and communicator, has come to be loved and respected by many who are interested in contact with the 'other worlds'. He has been in direct teaching communication with me for over thirty years, but I have known him as a 'companion' for the whole of my life.*

## HEALING

As part of his communications, Gildas gives teaching about healing. Specifically he speaks of the channelling of subtle energies through one person to another, in order to aid healing and growth. He makes it clear that healing is not just for obvious sickness, disease or disability but to help in raising our ceilings of potential. He maintains that healing should not be seen as a force directed solely to restoring a state of health which has previously been known. Full openness to the healing journey involves being taken through and beyond dis-ease into a new state of awareness and

*See *Gildas Communicates, Seven Inner Journeys, The Healing Spectrum* and *A Question of Guidance* (C. W. Daniel).

understanding of what it means to be whole and well. This may or may not be directly related to the wellness of the physical body. It encompasses spiritual understanding, a sense of purpose, emotional wellbeing and an ease and excitement at being alive.

This sort of healing is not a 'handing over' to a healer, therapist or doctor but is a consciously directed growth process. It may be assisted and guided by others but the aim is self-healing ability, awareness and self-responsibility. It is also about the early recognition of the factors which cause disease and thus about prevention as well as cure.

The acquisition of an awareness of an energy system long recognized in Eastern esoteric teaching as 'The Chakras' is a tool which helps in working with healing growth. When chakras are also understood as a 'Map of Consciousness' which helps our knowledge of who we are, whence we came and the nature of our individual and collective purpose, then the work takes on an even greater personal immediacy.

## CHAKRAS AND THE SUBTLE ENERGY FIELD OR 'AURA'

There is an energy field around every human being which is spiritually described and clairvoyantly perceived as the aura. This may be seen in colour or as a vague light. It may be sensed as private space or experienced as a subtle electrical tingling around an individual. The aura usually stretches about four to six inches (10 – 15 cm) out from the physical body. Once a person is truly dead there is no vitality in or around the physical body. The subtle energy field is no longer functioning, a vital essence has been withdrawn.

Those who are clairvoyantly gifted or who have trained their subtle sensitivity can describe the full radiant colours which constitute the auric field. Some colours remain constant while others change according to an individual's mood or state of physical, emotional, mental and spiritual health.

Much of the colour and energy of the auric field is supplied by the chakras. For anyone able to see or sense these, they are wheels of light and colour interpenetrating with, affecting and affected by the physical body. Most chakras carry links to specific parts of the glandular system and might therefore be described as subtle glands.

The word *chakrum* is Sanskrit and means 'wheel'. Properly speaking chakrum is the singular form and chakra the plural but in the west it is usual to speak of one chakra and many chakras, a practice I shall follow throughout this book.

Another Sanskrit word, *nadis*, refers to the lines of force forming intangible layers and networks of energy which are the main substance of subtle bodies which surround each one of us. The places where these lines or nadis are produced and at which they intersect, are the chakras. The 'major' chakras occur where many of these lines are produced and cross each other. 'Minor' chakras are formed where there are less busy production and crossing points.

The subtle energy field around each human being and living organism can be photographed by the process known as Kirlian photography. (See *Glossary*.) Diagnoses as to physical or emotional states can be made from these photographs.

If you want to experience contact with your own subtle energy field in a simple way, open and contract your hands a few times and then gradually bring your palms towards each other from a distance, until they are between four to six inches (10 – 15 cm) apart. As the energy field of each palm encounters the other you will sense a resistance or a slight tingling. There are 'echoes' of all the chakras in the palms of the hands. Flexing the hands awakens, or opens these chakras, sets their energy buzzing and enables you to experience your own subtle energy activity. Try it with a friend or partner, sensing the difference between their energy field and your own.

# NAMES AND LOCATIONS OF THE CHAKRAS

On page 5 the diagram shows the seven major chakras, plus the Alter Major, and their positions in relationship to the physical body. They are named in descending order as Crown, Brow, Alter Major, Throat, Heart, Solar Plexus, Sacral and Root. Semantic difficulties can arise simply because there is a variety of terminology, some of which is Eastern and some more Westernized. For instance different teachers use the terms 'Sacral', 'Hara' or 'Spleen' to refer to the chakra which is two fingers below the navel. Confusion of terminology around 'Brow', 'Ajna' or 'Third Eye' also occurs. Problems arise if these terms are used inter-changeably within the usual sevenfold system when minor or additional chakras come under discussion. Many channelled sources and gifted clairvoyant observers now speak of newly awakening chakras which are becoming a part of the major system. In Chapter 10 on new chakras, some of these are discussed and some terms which have previously been interchanged are used more specifically.

Most Eastern traditions describe a sevenfold major chakra system, at the same time acknowledging varying large numbers of minor chakras throughout the body. Alice Bailey (see *Bibliography*) spoke of an eighth major chakra, giving it the Latin name 'Alta Major'. This chakra is included as an important one but with the spelling 'Alter Major' meaning 'other' rather than 'higher' major.

The expanded major chakra system suggests a total of twelve major points to which we should direct attention in order to aid self-healing and growth. The number twelve is certainly important in other ways. We have twelve astro-logical signs, twelve calendar months in a year, and it is expected that twelve planets will eventually be discovered. Chakras have often been linked to planets and signs, making them the astrology and astronomy of the physical and subtle bodies.

An assumption may be made that the words 'higher' or 'lower' are terms of evaluation. When used to refer to

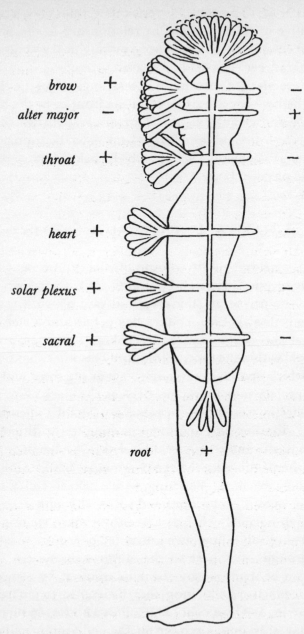

crown +

brow +                    −

alter major −             +

throat +                  −

heart +                   −

solar plexus +            −

sacral +                  −

root +

*The seven best-known chakras, plus the alter major. Energy flows from positive to negative*
*( + = positive polarity, − = negative polarity) and up and down the central column.*
*Note the reversed polarity of the alter major.*

chakras it is important to remember that they are only descriptive of their position in relationship to the physical body when upright. There is not a hierarchical system within the chakras, each is part of a team.

There is a lack of agreement in teachings about the chakras as to whether they are situated in the front or at the back of the body and its auric field. There are systems which place some at the front and some at the back. The diagram on page 5 attempts to depict the way in which chakras interpenetrate with the physical body.

## CHAKRA 'PETALS' AND 'STEMS'

There is a central subtle column of energy interpenetrating with the physical body and running from the crown of the head to the perineum (the area mid-way between the anus and the genitals). Each chakra has petals and a stem. The stems of the crown and root chakras are open and are contained within the central column. The other chakras have petals which open into the auric field at the front and stems which project into the auric field at the back. The stems normally stay closed but the petals are flexible, opening and closing, vibrating and turning according to the different life situations encountered. A healthy chakra is a flexible chakra. Where there is dis-ease the chakra energies become inflexible or actually blocked. Working with chakras can thus aid physical, mental, emotional and spiritual health.

Though normally closed, a healthy chakra stem is like a self-opening valve. It allows unwanted energy or reaction to pass through. It is part of the elimination system. These stems can be damaged by shock or trauma, by over-use of drugs (medical or hallucinogenic), by lengthy or too frequent anaesthesia, and by alcohol and tobacco abuse. In such cases they may stay open, rendering the individual vulnerable to outside influences of all kinds. This open state of the stems can be healed through an understanding of colour and energies and by the receiving of the sort of healing which can be channelled through the hands. Much chakra work, though, is of a self-help nature. With a little knowledge and practice you can do a great deal to change your life with exercises which are almost as straightforward as breathing or through creative and colourful visualization.

## CLEARING THE CENTRAL COLUMN

A first and most important exercise is for clearing your central column. Since each chakra feeds into and is fed from the central column, keeping it clear can help in balance, vitality and healing at all levels. The following simple exercises will effect this clearance. Chakra energy needs to move easily both upwards and downwards through your body. The exercises also help to establish this movement.

## TWO EXERCISES FOR INCREASED AWARENESS OF THE CENTRAL COLUMN AND ITS ENERGY FLOW

These are simple exercises, both based on the in-breath and the out-breath, one a straightforward breathing exercise, the other including visualization.

### 1. Non-Visual

Stand or sit with your spine straight and your body balanced. Do not cross your legs if you are sitting in a chair, or your ankles if you are sitting on the floor. (Lotus or 'cross-legged' posture excepted.)

Begin by being aware of the rhythm of your breathing and letting it slow down. You now draw the breath in as though it comes from just above the crown of your head: draw it down through the centre of your body; change to the out-breath at a point which feels natural for you and breathe out as though right down and through your legs and into the earth. (The breath will not go down through your legs if you are in a cross-legged or lotus position but these postures automatically balance energies in the body.) Breathe in this way about five times (i.e. five breath sequences: in/out = one sequence).

Now on the alternate breath sequence begin to breathe up from the earth, through the centre of your body, letting the out-breath go out through the crown of your head.

Continue to breathe in this way, without straining or forcing for about five minutes. Always end on the downward breath sequence, repeating it in this direction more than once if you wish. Feel the balance of your body and then continue with your normal tasks.

(You can also use this exercise as a preparation for meditation or before doing any of the other exercises in this book.)

## 2.   Visualization for the Central Column

If the outdoor conditions are favourable and there is a suitable tree that you know, it is good to do this exercise with your back against it and your bare feet on the earth. At other times follow the posture instructions as for exercise 1.

Begin by being aware of your breathing rhythm and let it steady and perhaps slow down a little.

Visualize yourself as a tree. Your branches stretch out above, your roots stretch deeply into the earth, your trunk is straight and strong. You are nurtured by the four elements. Sun (fire), warms you and air refreshes you. Your roots are in the earth and seek the underground streams and sources of living water.

Breathe in through your branches, from the elements of air and sun, take the breath right down through your trunk and breathe out strongly into your roots, into the earth and the streams of living water.

Breathe in now from the earth and the living water, bring the breath up through your roots, through your trunk, into your branches and breathe out into the elements of air and sun.

Repeat these two breath sequences for five to ten minutes. Then gradually let the visualization fade. Feel your feet firmly on the ground, your own space all around you and proceed with a sense of centredness to your normal activities.

## CHAKRA POLARITIES AND CORRESPONDENCES

With the exception of the alter major chakra (see page 128), the petals carry a positive and the stems a negative polarity (see diagram on page 5). Again, these terms are not evaluatory but are rather used in an electrical or magnetic sense. More explanation about polarity is given in Chapter 16 (see page 171 – 2).

A large part of life experience comes to us through the five senses – smell, taste, sight, touch, hearing. Our world is full of fragrances, tastes, colours, objects, textures and sounds. As we mature we accumulate a great deal of information about the delights and dangers of the world in which we live. The way in which we function as adults is affected by the positive and negative experiences we have had. The physical senses are powerful stimulants to mind and emotion. For instance, the smell and sound of chalk on a board will often evoke startlingly vivid memories of school. Such recall may be full of pleasure or pain according to our individual experience.

You will find a summary of these and other correspondences at the start of each chakra chapter.

## DEVELOPMENTAL STAGES

The new-born baby has its own complete aura and chakra system but the developmental stages through which we pass in life affect each of the first *five* chakras in turn – root, sacral, solar plexus, heart, throat. These are linked to each of the physical senses and to the basic elements from which life experiences come – earth, water, fire, air, ether or akasha. Every chakra produces and is affected by particular colours. Each one stores a range of life experience for us and also links to the physical functioning of our bodies. With a little patience and practice, working with the chakras can unlock a wealth of information about us. Unsuspected strengths or gifts will emerge and information essential to full physical and emotional healing will be revealed. Although the chakras other than the first five are not connected with a developmental stage or a sense it must always be remembered that the chakras are a team. They develop concurrently and each team member is affected by the strengths or weaknesses of the others.

## CHAKRA COLOURS

The original seven chakras carry the colours of the rainbow spectrum. This does not necessarily mean that they *are* those colours but that they are responsible for that colour note within your chakra team and auric field. Any colour may be 'seen' or sensed in *any* chakra. It could be said that each chakra has its own full spectrum of colour. The presence, quality and degree of other colours reflects information about ourselves. For further information on colours turn to the section 'Using the Colours for Healing' in Chapter 3 and pages 172 – 4 in Chapter 16, where there is information on the meaning of the colours.

## CHAKRAS AS A 'MAP OF CONSCIOUSNESS'

In moving into the more detailed descriptions of the chakras it will be seen that each is like a separate universe, though linked to all the different areas of life, growth and abilities. Though understanding them separately, awareness of the whole team must always be kept in mind. Chakras can be seen as a map of consciousness charting a spiritual and evolutionary journey, not only for the individual but for the whole of humanity.

Of the multitudinous impressions and experiences which bombard us every hour of every day only a very small proportion arc assimilated into full awareness. Many of us feel an urge to participate more fully, responsibly and excitingly in life's journey. We long to know ourselves better in every way. The self-understanding gained through contact with our chakras helps in making more dynamic, exciting but realistic life choices. The journey may be complex but it keeps alive a sense of wonder. Human potential is vast. There is no point at which 'all is done'; there are always new opportunities.

Consciousness is a progressive revelation. That which is unconscious is undefined, formless, dark, shadowy, without concept. In a state of health there is constant movement between the known and the unknown.

This is the context of this chakra map. The chakras are moving, vibrating, pulsating wheels of light. Connecting with them gives us a better understanding of ourselves and the way in which we relate to our partners and and all who are important in our lives. Parents can find a deeper awareness of the development, difficulties and needs of their children. Damage to the vulnerable inner child in each one of us can be healed. Every aspect of our functioning, expression and fulfilment in life can be better understood and therefore enhanced.

The chakra information presented here sometimes differs from that described by other sources or teachers. These differences are not intended to be contradictory. One of Gildas' earliest and most basic teachings is about the multi-faceted jewel of truth. The finite mind can never hold all the facets of truth at any one time. To try to do so is a limitation of truth, particularly in the spiritual field. Different systems are not necessarily in opposition to each other but need to be seen as complementary or amplificatory. Different teachers work from different perspectives but the aim must be to arrive at a place where truth becomes a personal and resonant experience.

Teaching is thus a 'leading out' – from the Latin *educare* – a structure to enable a journey; not a dogma to imprison or limit. Apparent inconsistencies can become creative opportunities, to motivate an inner relationship to personal truth, if the immediate desire for intellectual order and concurrence is relinquished.

## USING THIS BOOK

The information given in this book is not only about growth and healing but about life and its dilemmas. The teaching is an interpretation of ancient classical spiritual knowledge. It has been inspired not only by Gildas' discarnate guidance but has also grown from my experience in leading workshops and working as a counsellor and healer. Some information has come from Gildas' responses to questions posed by individuals and groups. The case histories are from my personal work with groups and with individual clients (names and some details have been changed to maintain confidentiality).

There is a chapter devoted to each of the seven main chakras moving from the root upwards. In the root chakra there is extra information, for example on how to work with fragrances, that you will need to refer to when working with the other chakras. After the seven main chakras there is discussion of the newly awakening or additional chakras, each of which has its own chapter. Following this is a chapter dealing with questions I'm frequently asked by clients or in workshops. These cover learning to sense the chakras, developing the ability to visualize, the meaning of the colours in the chakras, the use of massage and how to work with crystals. This information will be useful to you as you begin using the meditations and exercises given at the end of each chapter.

It is useful to keep a notebook or loose-leaf file as a record of your progress. Before you work with the guided visual meditations you may like to speak them on to a tape, so that you can listen to them rather than having to memorize all the stages.

I recommend that you should get at least a general idea of all the information in this book before you start to work specifically. As you read the case histories you may identify problems of your own and thus know the chakras on which you wish to focus. It is not necessary to work in any specific order, though the new chakras should be left until last. Do not concentrate on one chakra for months on end, always create a balance by working with its chakra pair (see page 178), or with the heart and root chakra as well. Do not spend longer than one hour each day in concentrated chakra work.

# Chapter 2

# A Personal Story

Since my introduction to chakras over thirty years ago, working with them has led me to a deeper understanding of personal growth. In times of difficulty, accident or illness I have enhanced my internal resources and accelerated healing by using the chakras as self-help tools.

My childhood, in the war years, was uneasy and deprived in many ways. There was an early awareness of being different from my parents and my brother; we had a mutual difficulty in living together. I was born with very little sight in my right eye. This was casually assumed to be a 'lazy' eye. I spent some years being forced to wear an eye patch over my good eye in order to make the 'naughty, lazy eye' work. It was not until I was eleven that it was discovered that the right eye was neither lazy nor naughty but physically incapable of much sight because of scarring on the retina. During a rapid growth period from age twelve to fourteen my left eye became more and more short-sighted. The specialist feared that I would soon be blind.

I had a passion for languages and I longed to study them at university. However, my eye-sight problem precluded reading or doing any close work by artificial light, so I was advised to take up gardening as a career. Finding this recommendation unacceptable, a compromise was reached and I found myself more or less pushed into what was considered to be a 'practical' training for teaching young children of nursery and infant-school age. I was terrified of children, confused about my eye-sight and bursting with a rich inner and dream life which I knew no one around me would understand. In thick glasses, ankle socks, my school uniform skirt and a pudding basin hair-cut, I arrived at college to begin my professional training.

Then the miracles began. In 1956 I was at the only college in England to have a student-counselling service. My tutor persuaded me to see Dr Swainson, a pioneer student counsellor and Jungian therapist, who also had a long association with The White Eagle Lodge. It took a while for me to realize that this gentle woman could be trusted with my innermost thoughts, fears, hopes, dreams and experiences. My inner world became validated. Self-respect began to grow. My eyesight quickly stabilized and then improved. Most important the 'being' whose presence I had sensed near me since childhood was identified as 'Gildas' my discarnate guide, teacher and friend. Reassured that I was not after all, going mad, I could allow Gildas' communications to flow and develop.

Reconciling myself to teaching, I taught in Infants' Schools for over twenty years. I married, had a daughter and divorced. As a single parent, teaching was a very useful career. When my daughter was old enough for me to take some risks, I retrained as a counsellor and gradually set up a private practice which today includes counselling, channelling, healing, lecturing, running workshops, travelling and writing.

Learning to use the benefits of chakra knowledge to help myself in times of change, stress or crisis was a gradual process. Realizing how chakra work can enhance each day has been a joy. Out of my own experience and Gildas' teaching have emerged the tools and insights with which to help others. By describing my own journey to you as a chakra case history I can perhaps be more explicit.

Our early environment affects the development of the chakras. Severe confrontations or deprivations will block the ability of the chakras to work for us at every level of our health and wellbeing. Lesser confrontations or challenges may give extra impetus to the development of chakra strengths, like a plant, which pruned, grows stronger. The well-nurtured or developed chakra will fortify our life-strengths. In areas where certain abilities are lacking or have been inhibited, the chakras become blocked, under-active, over-active, closed, too open, too pale or over-intense in their colours.

The earliest years affect the root and sacral chakras. My childhood was beset by a lack of bonding with my parents. We had little in common. At a physical level there were all the deprivations of a war-time childhood. I was often humiliated or given severe physical punishments. In another sense, however, my parents were good providers. They put a priority on a warm and comfortable home, materially speaking. Money was always short but ingenuity was strong. Part of my early years were spent in Bournville, the garden suburb of Birmingham, which was then on the edge of the countryside. Natural beauty was never far away. My father was a Conscientious Objector but was given war-work in caring for evacuees at a large requisitioned house and farm in the Warwickshire countryside. Some of the older evacuees gave me a taste of the emotional warmth which my parents were unable to provide. There were animals, trees, flowers and all the privileges of country living.

The root chakra helps in developing the ability to be fully here and present on earth and in the material world. Psychologists and counsellors today recognize that the healthy adult needs self-nurturing abilities. This includes: claiming and creating a congenial living space; being able to take 'time out'; having a sound balance between acknowledging personal needs and those of others; taking pleasure and pride in looking after our bodies; eating in a wholesome way with enjoyment; handling money and the material world with equilibrium and also enjoying animals and the world of nature.

These positive environmental factors have given me a relatively well-functioning root chakra. There can be 'wobbly bits' around food and money and I have a tendency to be a 'workaholic'. Meditating on my root chakra, breathing into it to aid its flexibility and visualizing its healthy colours help me in overcoming these problems when they arise.

The privations and conflicts of my childhood have shown up most in my sacral, solar plexus, heart and throat chakras. Too many restrictive boundaries and lack of 'permission' to be myself have meant a long struggle to recognize and claim my own 'power' and to know who I am. Empowerment is one of the sacral chakra issues; identity belongs to the solar plexus. It was strange that my parents chose to push me in the direction of teaching. The 'voice' of my own being had been so denied and severely repressed that severe shyness made me almost unable to commune with others. It took a lot of work with my throat chakra before my ability to communicate became free. I recognize now that I *am* a teacher but the road to that recognition has been long and hard.

The sacral chakra also affects relationship abilities, including sexuality. My marriage broke down because my husband and I were incompatible on almost every level. Until I worked with my sacral chakra I did not recognize what incompatibility meant. I thought that I was always wrong and had to change and adapt to suit everyone else. I too easily accepted blame and the wrong sort of responsibility. I was a willing 'hook' for many projections. Not only my sexuality but my creativity were blocked. My 'true self' loves colour. Although my first home after divorce was comfortable and warm (root chakra), most things in it were dull brown. Where I used colour in that house, it was garish, unsubtle and disharmonious. I dressed myself in browns, fawns and navies, which do nothing at all for my particular colouring. Establishing a stronger flow between my sacral and throat chakras has helped to change all this.

The solar plexus chakra affects and is affected by identity crises. I needed skilled help in these areas and my solar plexus chakra is now quite strong. I work with it directly when issues of identity and self-assertion challenge or confront. At a physical level the solar plexus affects eyesight. Mine began to improve when my identity issues received help. Visualizing pure golden sunlight flooding into this chakra helps me to clearer vision in every sense of the word. In particular, I feel it has been a major help in keeping my physical eyesight stable even through the vulnerable menopausal life phase.

The heart chakra has a connection to the physical sense of touch. It affects the development of compassion and empathy, but also of healthy detachment. The quality of one's relationship to religion partly belongs to the heart and partly to the throat. A blocked or under-developed heart chakra can cause confusion, inconsistency or over-intensity.

Chakra blockages can lead to *over* or *under* reaction. In my case, the lack of physical bonding to my mother and an invasive quality which was present throughout my early years led to an over-sensitivity about physical contact with others. I retreated from any touching and distanced myself from people. I was confused about compassion and empathy. Sometimes a complete over-involvement in others' sufferings was physically painful or I would feel suffocated. At other times I was so detached as not even to notice and thus, no doubt, seemed hard and unfeeling. Such fluctuations were not easy for my daughter in her upbringing. In my later teenage years I was passionately and narrowly religious and judgemental. Work with my heart chakra enabled me to be more open towards others without negative vulnerability, and also to leave behind rigid dogma and seek my own inner spiritual truth.

When healing and improving ourselves, the chakras

change and respond even without consciously working with them. The advantage in the direct approach to them is one of speed, efficiency and economy in effecting change. Growth may be said to be a way of life; many psychotherapeutic approaches take years to show results and are only available to a privileged few. Chakra work does not necessarily replace other therapies but is a safe self-help tool which brings swift and tangible results. It can thus shorten and deepen other therapeutic interventions and be invaluable in maintaining any progress which has been achieved.

In this, my own brief case history I have endeavoured to indicate how life-happenings affect the chakra energies. In the following pages each chakra is explored in detail and case histories are given.

As you read the case histories in each chapter consider your own life pattern and the areas in which you feel most wounded, stressed or under-developed. The developmental age is a good guide. If any of the case histories tell a story which particularly moves you, read all the information about that chakra with extra care. If you identify yourself with several of the statements made, then this could be the chakra requiring the most immediate attention. Don't worry if you pick out something in each case history or problem area – the tendency to 'acquire' all the symptoms we read about is well known! Try marking the extent of your identification with each chakra on a five point scale, using 'five' as the score showing the most need for that chakra to be healed or developed and 'one' as the score for the least need. Practical instructions and suggestions for chakra work are given at the end of each chapter.

# Chapter 3

# The Root Chakra

**Location** Perineum (The area mid-way between the anus and the genitals. The petals face downwards, between the legs, the stem faces upwards into the central column and is naturally and healthily slightly open.)

**Key Words** Rootedness, Incarnation, Acceptance, Self-Preservation, Concept

**Developmental Age** 0–3/5 years

**Colours** Red, Brown and Mauve

**Element** Earth

**Sense** Smell

**Body** Physical

**Glandular Connection** Gonads

**Quietening Fragrances** Cedarwood, Patchouli

**Stimulating Fragrances** Musk, Lavender, Hyacinth

**Crystals and Gemstones** Smoky Quartz, Garnet, Alexandrite, Ruby, Agate, Bloodstone, Onyx, Tiger's Eye, Rose Quartz

## Prayer or Affirmation

Through incarnation may spirit be brought into matter. Through rootedness may life force be recharged and exchanged. We acknowledge wholeness and seek to gain and to reflect acceptance.

## Root Chakra Case History

Martin came to me for counselling. He was a married man
with three young children. His wife had her own career
before the children were born. Externally Martin was
doing well. He was climbing the executive ladder. The
family had a lovely home in the commuter belt. He
seemed proud of the fact that Janet, his wife, did not need
to work and could therefore devote her time to the home
and children. Janet was content to be taking some years
out of her career and was enjoying being a mother without
the stress of other work. They had no money worries.

Internally Martin felt stressed. His relationship with
Janet was undergoing pressures which he found difficult to
define. He had increasing periods of deep depression. He
loved his children but life was becoming devoid of any fun
or joy. He was unable to play or show real affection. His
sexual drive was diminishing. In his spare time Martin
worked hard at home-maintenance and improvement
jobs. He complained that he never had any time to
himself.

As the counselling progressed it became clear that
Martin was driving himself to be the traditional 'good
provider'. His own parents had been curiously
uninterested in him as a child. They both had careers. It
had been a 'nice' home, but one which lacked warmth and
'comfortable clutter'. An only son, he had never really
been a child. As he got more in touch with his feelings,
extreme anguish about the loneliness of his childhood
produced tears and anger. Early bonding with his mother
had not been good and real closeness, with either parent,
had never been developed. It was a sterile picture. Now, in
his own marriage, he was over-compensating. He was
trying very hard to give his children the childhood he had
never had. To some extent it was working but the cost to
his own wellbeing was increasing. He had lacked all the
things which help to make a healthy root chakra, and

therefore was unable to be relaxed about providing them for others. He was doing everything from a place of will and control in himself, rather than from natural warmth. The pressures in his relationship with Janet had developed because increasingly, in emotional ways, he was tending to become one of the children, competing for love. This left Janet feeling very alone in her parenting in a manner which was difficult to define since, in so many ways, Martin was such a model husband and father.

Obviously Martin had to work psychologically to deal with his own unnourished inner child and to improve his self-image. He agreed also to work with his chakras, concentrating particularly on the root. He did this mainly through using the techniques suggested at the end of this chapter. The chakra work supported and deepened the psychological work. Within a relatively short time his sense of fun returned. He began to play more with his children, fully realizing that he was doing so partly to replace play opportunities which had never existed for him. He became more able to nurture himself without demanding this in emotionally complicated ways from Janet. He rediscovered a love of drawing, painting and the study of art. His sexual energy returned.

Although creativity and sexuality can be the province of the sacral chakra, in Martin's case the root chakra was most important because it was undeveloped and blocked. There were insufficient energy currents to flow upwards into the sacral chakra. When the root was stronger, the sacral also became more colourful and energized without Martin needing to work as intensively with it as he did for the root chakra.

# THE KEY WORDS

## Rootedness

This is in some ways synonymous with 'grounding'. In accepting incarnation we become rooted into the element of earth and more consciously interactive with the life of the planet. The more we are rooted the less does life on earth become a burden. Difficulties take on a new perspective, giving us more over-all purpose and sense of meaning.

## Incarnation and Acceptance

The Concise Oxford Dictionary defines incarnation as 'embodiment in flesh'. This needs to be *accepted* before we can become grounded or *rooted*. The key words speak for each other and are inseparable.

Much esoteric spiritual teaching presupposes an acceptance of reincarnation and many lifetimes. Such teaching includes the belief that we choose the parents to whom we will be born, the historical time, the culture and our position within it. These choices reflect the reasons and purposes for our incarnation. Making the reasons more conscious is part of the pattern of life. Some of this information about life choices and purpose is imprinted into the energy field and colour patterns of the root chakra.

## Self-Preservation

This links the root chakra to all instinctual behaviour. Through instinct we preserve ourselves from danger. We learn, for instance, that we can use fire for warmth and cooking, but that it has to be contained and controlled in order to stop it from injuring us or being destructive.

Fears which warn us to stay within certain limitations are mechanisms of self-preservation. Fear of falling is one. Some of the competitive areas of life, particularly in the sports world, lead us to test the boundaries between self-preservation and danger. There is a thrill in testing ourselves in this way. As young children explore the world, they should be discouraged from becoming physically competitive too soon. On the other hand they should not be over-inhibited by parental anxiety. Children climbing, for instance, will not usually over-extend their capacities unless they are given the idea that it would be 'brave' to climb at least as high as a more naturally confident and coordinated friend. Equally, over-restraint of adventurous children will make them unsure of their own instinctual judgements. They may either become too dependent on the judgement of others or be defiant and go beyond their own limitations, always too high and too close to the edge. Strengthening the root chakra rebalances instinctual judgement.

## Concept

In the section on developmental age it will be seen that proper play opportunities for children lay the foundations for the forming of concepts firmly derived from experience. Concepts are necessary to the abstract thinking which is an ingredient of creativity. This key-word illustrates that good grounding is the foundation for the development of the fullest potential possible in each individual.

People who have difficulty with conceptual thought may be lacking in early play experiences. Fortunately it is rarely too late to learn to play or to get other insights which help to heal the wounds of early experience and the 'inner child' which resides in each one of us.

## THE DEVELOPMENTAL AGE

For this chakra, it is from birth to three to five years. Young children develop more quickly now than, say, twenty-five years ago, hence the variation in the upper age range. The age range for each chakra does not mean that it stops developing after this period or that the other chakras are non-existent at this time. There are particular phases of early life which are crucial to each of the first five chakras. If the needs of each stage are well met, the chakra will function more easily, strongly and openly in every other life-phase. If the needs are neglected, then the chakra becomes an important focus for diagnosis and healing whenever physical illnesses or emotional and psychological difficulties manifest.

The early years are foundations for the rest of life. The degree to which the primary needs – such as warmth, food, shelter and love – are met, will reflect into the development and health of the chakra.

The key words of the root chakra are particularly related to the developmental age. This is a pre-conceptual phase, yet a vital exploration of the world is taking place. Language is being learned from the moment of birth. A rich variety of play opportunities is essential. It behoves us to remember that what may easily be dismissed as 'play' is, in fact, serious *work* for the young child.

The Swiss psychologist and educationalist, Jean Piaget, studied the relationship of a child's experience to the formation of true concepts. When a child crawls and first begins to walk it registers experiences of size and area. Later activities such as painting on varying sizes of paper with large and small brushes provide for an extension of this exploration. Without a variety of such experiences there can be no real concept of size and area. The subsequent learning of mathematical formulae must link to direct experience. Dealing with colours, sorting and matching, putting together jigsaw puzzles, all give the basic skills required for literacy and numeracy. A very young child may recite numbers and appear to count but only time and experience brings the recognition that five beads in a box remain five and that when two more are put with them it is possible to 'count on', not needing to start the counting process over again from 'one'. This knowledge is called 'conservation of number'. Learning to differentiate shapes is a prerequisite to being able to recognize words and letters on a page. An optimum amount of experience at the pre-conceptual stage forms the basis for the full development of innate intelligence.

Playing with water and observing how a certain quantity looks in a narrow bottle and then how the same quantity looks in a wide bottle; moving heavy and light loads of dry sand and wet sand or wooden bricks in buckets, plastic delivery lorries, or other containers, lead to more understanding of the conservation and the nature of matter. The possibilities are immense. Children of this age must climb, touch, feel, squeeze, hear, taste, smell and observe their surroundings. These experiences are not only necessary for the development of understanding about life but also to rooting into and accepting incarnation.

The quality of 'play' opportunities reflects the freedoms and boundaries which can be provided in a given environment. Opportunity or freedom to explore is only one aspect. There must also be boundaries which are neither too rigid nor too loose and permissive. Extremes in both directions can lead to anxieties and insecurities. The parents' role in establishing the quality of guidance and protection offered to a child is never an easy one. Parents who are too anxious, strict or over-protective may cause a child to be either fearful or rebellious. Where too little guidance is given a child may feel insecure, 'unheld' and unloved. There are no categoric rules to help in finding the balanced position. All children are individuals and their needs vary.

It is not my intention to present a child-care manual, but these are important issues that affect the root chakra. Parents can do much to help the rootedness and incarnation of their children. Emphasis is laid nowadays on preparation for parenthood. This should include looking at ways in which parents might heal their own root chakra wounding so that children may have optimum early opportunities. It is almost standard that in healing the root chakra, a need for greater self-nourishment and changing attitudes will emerge. As Martin found, knowing how much had been missed in his childhood gave practical pointers for the sort of activities which could help the healing process in himself.

No environment is without its traumas, blockages and challenges. *Enough* of what is needed at each stage results in an overall healthiness and zest for life. Colourful and pulsating chakras sustain vitality and open opportunities.

## THE COLOURS

Red is the essential or basic colour for the root chakra. This colour has the lowest vibrational rate in the colour spectrum. The root chakra is responsible for producing the colour red in our energy field. A healthy energy field is one which contains some of each colour of the spectrum. The distribution of the colours reflect individual gifts and talents. Aura readers interpret the colours and their distribution in order to give the information which the sitter may be seeking. When healthy, the root chakra produces and distributes red light and vitality. If you have difficulty with any root chakra issues, colour visualization is a powerful aid to self-healing. Brown and mauve are also produced by the root chakra and can be used in healing for it and any of the life areas which affect and are affected by the state of the root.

## USING THE COLOURS FOR HEALING

Although a healthy root chakra may clairvoyantly be seen to produce quite brilliant reds, in healing work the brightest shades should be used with discretion. The simplest and most effective visual healing exercise for each chakra is to imagine the 'home' colours of the chakra flowing into the petals to feed it. At the root, however, softer colours of the red range should be used, as brilliant reds can be too challenging or over-stimulating. Warm, deep rose colours are best. When working with a particular chakra you can try wearing clothes of its colour range, or putting appropriately coloured objects into your living environment. This enables touches of the

brighter reds and carmines to be used beneficially but
without over-intense effects.

If you have a resistance to reds use the browns and mauves,
or try green instead. Each colour has its 'complement' and
green is the complement of red. If you stare hard at something
red for a few moments and then close your eyes you will see
green as an 'after image'. These colours are interdependent
and in healing can literally be used to complement or sub-
stitute for each other.

As you practise the exercises your sensitivity will increase
and you may become very aware of the colour activity in
your chakras. Never forget that any colour can appear in any
chakra with positive meaning. When you are visualizing
colours for healing try to see them as vibrant and translucent
like the colours in stained glass when sunlight is passing
through it. If you sense that some of the colours in your
chakras are dense or opaque this could indicate areas which
require attention or things which are beginning to emerge
into fuller consciousness. With colour or energy 'experiences' and observations in the chakras, nothing is 'wrong'.
Even black has its place. How and where the colour is
presenting itself gives useful information and feedback.
There is further information on the meaning of colours in the
chakras in Chapter 16.


# THE ELEMENT

In the visual breathing exercise given on pages 8 – 9, you are
asked to visualize the strong roots of a tree, deep in the earth,
seeking the nourishment of the earth itself and the streams of
living water which run through it.

Earth is dense physical matter. It is the 'plane' of which we
are most conscious. It is the substance which we use and
adapt to ensure our nourishment, shelter and many other
aspects of physical comfort.

Some spiritual teaching implies that we should despise

matter and seek only spiritual perfection. Death is seen as a 'release' and any subsequent existence as particularly joyful *because* of the freedom from bodily and material chains. Yet all around us there is evidence that earth is beautiful and wondrous, a living and continuous example of the miracle of creation. Our bodies are no less wondrous in their functioning. When we stop despising matter and putting it in negative polarity to the spiritual, then we truly begin to live a balanced life and encompass the possibility of joy. When we have a healthy respect for earth we live in greater harmony not only with our bodies but with the nature of earth itself.

It may be true that we can become trapped by matter in a different sense, if it is seen as the *only* reality. Confusion about the definition of reality, and confinement of it to that which is solid and tangible, can lead us indeed into illusion. Knowledge of different *levels* and manifestations of reality is essential to a truly spiritual journey. Setting up oppositions between that which is imaginary, illusory or ethereal and that which is real serves no useful purpose. Every level has its *own* reality.

The things of earth have long been things of great inspiration. Poets, artists, mystics and musicians have revelled not only in its beauties but in its incongruities and its sometimes ugly or comic juxtapositions. Great acts of sacrifice have been brought about by human compassion for those who are sick in body, lack shelter or are materially underprivileged. The energy-giving presence of an eternal sense of wonder is fed by the beauty of a flower, the curve of a contour, the rhythms of day and night, sun and moon, time and tide.

Many of our ancestors and some of the so-called pagan religions have been concerned with the privilege of life, with understanding earth, its rhythms and promise of abundance and manifestation. In our times the message is slowly coming through that our planet is being threatened, poisoned and polluted by our lack of respect for it. If the earth dies humankind dies with it.

One of the beneficial effects of such shocking knowledge may be to bring back a realization of the wonder of creation, the miracle of the life force, the sacredness of earth and the spirit resident in matter. Contact with and understanding of the root chakra brings the awareness that extension of consciousness is not only about moving upward and out of the body and matter. It is also about knowing and working with the wider dimensions of the material world in which we live. Spiritual living is about being effective and congruent in the world as we know it, as well as about exploring other dimensions. To be too grounded can diminish horizons; to be too ethereal makes a nonsense of the personal and collective purposes of incarnation.

## THE SENSE

This is the first sense experienced by the newly-born child. It affects and enables the ability to connect and bond with the mother. Smell leads the new-born to the breast and triggers the instinct to suckle. If the mother does not smell right, the breast may be rejected thus causing early feeding and bonding difficulties.

People can actively smell danger. Animals smell, and are made nervous by, the release of adrenalin in humans who are afraid of them. Smell triggers the 'fight or flight' mechanism, in which the smell of danger causes an autonomous release of adrenalin into the blood stream giving extra strength if we have to fight, extra speed if we need to retreat and quickening all reaction times.

In our deodorized society we are losing touch with natural smells and the instincts which they arouse. Yet research shows that smell is a powerful element in sexual attraction between human beings. The very latest work on pheromones is expected to lead to a breakthrough in helping people with sexual difficulties.

Sex is connected to the root chakra only in so far as it is instinctual. The more conscious areas of sexuality belong rather to the sacral chakra.

## CHAKRAS, VIBRATIONAL RATES AND SUBTLE BODIES

The root is the *first* chakra. In Eastern teaching it is given the name 'Muladahara', meaning root or support. It is described as having four petals. Each subsequent chakra has an increasing number of petals until the crown is described as 'the thousand petalled lotus'.

The number of petals classically assigned to a chakra reflects the vibrational rate. Dense matter vibrates at a comparatively low speed and we experience it as solid. The electrical or magnetic energies which make up the auric field consist of interpenetrating layers of increasing vibrational rate. Each of these layers is connected to a chakra. A lower speed gives a simpler or more tangible feeling of movement. A higher speed gives a sense of uninterrupted flow of movement and of intangibility or complexity of form.

The term 'subtle bodies' is used to describe the intangible layers of energy which surround and interpenetrate with our physical substance. Traditionally there are seven subtle bodies and when we enter altered states of consciousness, for instance when meditating or dreaming, the experience takes place in – and is registered by – these other vibrational layers or bodies. They form the major part of what is known as the 'auric field'. Sensitivity training enables a greater awareness of our subtle bodies and subtle or auric energy field.

The root chakra has the lowest vibrational rate. It affects, and is most affected by, the physical body.

## RELATIONSHIP OF THE ROOT CHAKRA TO THE PHYSICAL BODY

Every chakra affects and is affected by the physical body and its health and functioning. This connection is particularly related to the glandular systems. Every chakra, except the root, also connects to a 'subtle body'. The root chakra, with its lowest vibrational rate, is the chakra of matter and is linked to the most solid aspects of the physical body such as bones, flesh, muscles and sinews. When there are disharmonies or disease in these parts the origins may be traced back to matters connected with the root chakra. Working with its colours, fragrances, crystals and the related psychological and emotional matters, will therefore help in healing these parts and also diseases such as rheumatism, osteo-arthritis, 'widow's hump', other bone diseases and cancers of bone, tissue and skin.

Learning to love our bodies more and to accept their challenges and limitations as well as their advantages and skills is an important factor in self-esteem and physical healing. If these things are difficult for you, working with the root chakra will help.

## THE GLANDULAR CONNECTION

The gonads are the glandular connection for the root chakra. They are the testes in men and the ovaries in women. They are part of the endocrine system, secretory cells with neighbouring capillaries linked by connective tissue. The pituitary gland is sometimes called the 'master gland'. It might be seen as the conductor of the glandular orchestra. At its 'command' hormones are secreted from the testes or ovaries. There is an obvious connection here to fertility and sexual functioning, drives and instincts. Secretions from the gonads ensure that the natural processes – such as puberty – happen as a matter of course and at the appropriate time.

Where there is dysfunction in these aspects of growth, specific work with the root chakra will again be of help in the healing process.

## WORKING WITH THE FRAGRANCES

Essential oils, which are pure plant and flower extracts, are being increasingly used for their therapeutic values for illness or stress. They have preventative as well as curative benefits. Even a subtle presence of the right blend of oils in an environment or on the body can help to minimise negative reactions to atmospheric pollution and to relieve stress and tension. Nurses are finding fragrances useful in aiding the recovery of patients in intensive care units.

Fragrances or oils for the chakras are classified under the headings of 'stimulating' or 'quietening'. As you learn to 'read' your chakras you may get a sense of under or over-activity. An over-active chakra feels excited and tingly or tense when attention is focused into it. Such a chakra may also be open and vulnerable. An under-active chakra may feel 'cold' or closed. It will be difficult to sense a response from it. Any images associated with it may be of closed flowers, closed doors, shields or defensive weapons.

As you open your awareness to the chakras you will find that insights about them permeate your full consciousness. You do not have to be gifted to 'sense' or 'see' subtle energies. In Chapter 16 there is more information about development of sensitivity and visualization, but having reached this point in reading about the root chakra, you may already have some ideas about whether yours is under-active, over-active or balanced. Use of the appropriate fragrances can help to adjust balances and to awaken closed chakras. If you want to feel calmer about the material world, your body or your incarnation, then the quietening fragrances of cedarwood or patchouli can be successfully used at your root chakra. If you want to be more stimulated to deal with these issues, more positively alive and vital, then the stimulating fragrances – musk, lavender and hyacinth – will help. If you are uncertain, then mix a little of each of the oils together to form a personal, root chakra balancing fragrance.

Some fragrances affect more than one chakra and while, for instance, patchouli is quietening for the root, it is stimulating for the throat. This means that when using the fragrance your intention, or purpose, must be absolutely clear. When the intention *is* clear, the fragrance will help towards the end to which it has been directed.

There are a number of ways in which the fragrances can be used. Put a few drops into your bath, heat it in a diffuser, burn it as a joss stick or incense. Sniff a few drops of oil from your hand or from cotton wool or apply it directly to the corresponding body area for the chakra, massage yourself with fragranced oil, or better still, get someone to do it for you. Most essential oils are very concentrated, so that when applying them straight on to the skin it is safer to put them into a gentler and more neutral 'carrying' oil such as almond or apricot kernel oil, or non-fragranced massage oil.

When using a diffuser, which means that the fragrances will permeate a room or house, it is important to obtain the type of diffuser which contains water. In these, the water, into which you pour a few drops of oil, is heated by a small candle or night-light. The oil itself is thus not burned directly. Over-direct heat changes the character of an oil and may alter the fragrance and its benefits.

It is great fun to experiment with mixing the fragrances to form a blended oil for the objective you have in mind. In this way you can create your individual fragrances and know that by wearing them a particular healing or growth process is being encouraged.

Firm body massage, with or without accompanying fragrances, is very helpful to the root chakra and to help in feeling more fully 'in' your body. Lighter or etheric forms of massage, which can also be accompanied by the use of oils, do not work so directly for the root chakra but are helpful for chakras above the solar plexus. See Chapter 16 for more information on massage and the chakras.

## THE CRYSTALS AND GEMSTONES

The main guideline in relating crystals to chakras, is colour. Dark stones and red stones are particularly related to the root because they have strong earthing or regenerative qualities. Chapter 16 gives more information about crystals and how to use them for self-healing.

☆ *Smoky Quartz* promotes calmness, centredness and groundedness. It helps to calm fear, panic or shock.

☆ *Garnet and Alexandrite* are regenerative and help flesh and tissue to heal. They bring comfort to the bereaved and help generally in all times of loss or change.

☆ *Ruby* vitalizes, nourishes and warms. It is the stone to use for healing when there has been a difficult birth or bonding to the mother has been delayed for some reason.

☆ *Agate* strengthens our sense of purpose and brings a *joie de vivre*. It is helpful to those who fear poverty and deprivation, as it encourages abundance. Agates help in the process of balancing the inner masculine and feminine energies. They are beneficial to those preparing and hoping for parenthood and to those who are already parents of growing children.

☆ *Bloodstone* is purifying. It helps blood disorders. Also use it if you want to acquire the practical and material skills which are needed these days.

☆ *Onyx* gives strength and stamina. It is a good stone for those who feel over-burdened by worldly responsibilities.

☆ *Tiger's Eye* enhances creativity. It is a stone of fertility, unity and strength. It is protective in times of danger and helpful when there are challenges to be met.

☆ *Rose Quartz* can be used for all chakras. At the root it encourages self-nurturing. It brings the quality of warm, unconditional, motherly love and helps to heal all who have had too little of this in their lives.

## MEDITATIONS AND SUGGESTIONS FOR WORKING WITH YOUR ROOT CHAKRA

Key words, element, sense, developmental age, colours, fragrances and crystals all help in arriving at a clearer understanding of the root chakra. The following exercises give more specific ways of working with it and there is more about visualization, meditation and sensitivity in Chapter 16 which it would be helpful to read before trying the exercises.

### 1.   Contacting and Sensing the Root Chakra

With practice this meditative exercise will develop your sensitivity and enable you to keep a check on the condition of your root chakra. Before starting, check the diagram on page 5. Note that the root chakra's petals are facing down from between your legs into the earth and its stem is facing upwards into the central energy column.

You will need paper and crayons, as drawing in colour is a part of this exploration. Make sure that you will be undisturbed and that you are comfortable. Sit in a chair or on the floor, or lie down. Let your body be symmetrical, don't cross your legs at knees or ankles. (A completely cross-legged or lotus posture is good, but only if you can manage either easily.)

Close your eyes ... be in touch with the rhythm of your breathing ... let that rhythm gradually help you focus your

attention into the bodily area of your root chakra ...
remember the positioning of the chakra, its petals and
stem ... sense the energy field of your root chakra ...
become aware of its movement ... its vibrancy ... its
undulation and turning .... Through breathing deeply into
the chakra area you may begin to get a sense of its colours or
of energies which could be expressed as colour .... Spend
about ten minutes using your breath to help you maintain
focus into your root chakra and when you feel ready, keeping
the quiet, meditative space around you, try to express what
you are feeling about your root chakra in colour on your
paper .... When you have finished exploring and drawing,
visualize the petals of the chakra, which will have opened up
for this exploration, closing in a little, not tightly or
completely, but just as part of the process of returning your
consciousness to where it needs to be for following your
everyday concerns. Finally visualize a cross of light in a circle
of light over the chakra. This should be an equal-armed
cross, or you can use a star of light in a circle of light if you
prefer.

## 2.   Images and Symbols

Repeat the above meditation, but instead of focusing on the
energy feeling of your chakra, see whether there is any
image, symbol, memory, fragrance or sound which comes to
you as you are in contact with your root. (Any or all of these.)
Close the petals and visualize the cross or star in the circle of
light at the end.

## 3.   Guided Visual Meditation for Your Root Chakra

Let your body be comfortable, relaxed and symmetrical
... be in touch with the rhythm of your breathing ...
centre into your own inner space and silence .... Visualize
yourself as a tree ... be aware of the whole tree and of what
sort of tree it is ... be particularly aware of its roots, going
down and spreading out into the earth ... feel the texture of
the earth and sense the roots drawing nourishment from it for

the tree ... be aware of the life-force of the tree ... the flows and currents within it ... sense the variation these might have with each season of the year ... more vital in spring ... slower and more contained in winter ... sense the cycle of its leaves, seeds, flowers and fruits ... (spend five to ten minutes on this first part of the meditation). Among the roots there is a special root called the tap root ... let your awareness be in the tap root ... experience there the memory of the tree's experience ... its first seeding, rooting and shooting ... its blending with and dependency upon the elements ... all the cycles of growth it has known ... be aware of a deep red colour in the centre of the tap root and of mauve around it ... be aware of the brown-ness of the earth ... and the warmth of the sun penetrating through it ... the comfort of water and air in the earth enable growth ... (five to ten minutes) ... sense a gentle throb in the tap root, like a heart beat and through that rhythm gradually connect with your own heart beat rhythm, the sense of your breathing, your body on the chair or floor ... return to your everyday surroundings. Put a cross of light in a circle of light over your root chakra and visualize a cloak of white light with a hood right around you. Feel the contact of your feet with the ground as you fully return.

## 4. Questions

Contemplate the questions: 'How do I smell the world?' 'How does the world smell me?'

## 5. Fragrances

As a result of the information you have now noted about yourself, choose the root chakra fragrance(s) which you would most like to work with. Use these in your environment or in your bath. Give yourself a leg and foot massage. Ask a friend or partner to massage the whole of you, gently but firmly defining your outline. See pages 33 – 5 for further directions and suggestions for working with fragrances.

## 6. Colours

Use the technique of 'breathing' into your root chakra, and 'feed' it with the colours given on page 20, though modifying the red to a strong rosy red. Remember to visualize the colours as translucent, like stained glass appears when sunlight passes through it. Close down the petals and visualize the cross or star in the circle of light to finish.

## 7. Getting in Touch with Your Incarnational Choices

Think about the circumstances of your birth and what it meant to your parents and family when you came into being. Consider the reasons why you may have chosen your particular parents, cultural heritage, place in society and historical time for this incarnation.

## 8. The Prayer or Affirmation

Meditate and reflect on the words given on page 20.

# Chapter 4

# The Sacral Chakra

**Location**  The petals are approximately two fingers below the navel. The stem corresponds to the sacrum area of the spine.

**Key Words**  Security, Sense of Others, Sexuality, Creativity, Empowerment, Co-creativity, Sincerity

**Developmental Age**  3/5–8 years

**Colours**  Orange, Amber, Gold

**Element**  Water

**Sense**  Taste

**Body**  Etheric

**Glandular Connection**  Lymphatics

**Quietening Fragrances**  Musk, Amber

**Stimulating Fragrances**  Rosemary, Rose Geranium

**Crystals and Gemstones**  Amber, Citrine, Topaz, Aventurine, Moonstone, Jasper

### Prayer or Affirmation

May the unity of humanity with each other and the earth enable true creativity. May release from a sense of sin and unworthiness lead us into the full knowledge of our empowerment as co-creators, at one with, and a part of God.

## Sacral Chakra Case History

Celia attended a number of my workshops on chakras and related themes. She is very gifted; skilled in art, calligraphy, woodwork and sewing, and also musically at home with the piano, violin and clarinet. She writes poetry and composes and writes lyrics for her own songs. Her technical ability in all these areas is outstanding. Her creative flair is inspirational. Yet Celia herself described her life as 'a shambles'. Aged thirty-five, she felt ashamed to be living on state benefits and was constantly moving from one inadequate bed-sit or flatlet to another. Her clothes were unflattering, her hair lifeless and her vitality low. Through the workshops I gradually got to know Celia well. She confided to me that she deliberately made herself unattractive because although she secretly longed for a loving relationship, she was afraid of commitment. Her scanty and inevitably brief sexual encounters had been emotionally and physically painful. Before closing down on this area of her life, she had challenged herself to experiment with relationships with women as well as men. With no experience of fulfilment, she now felt unclear about her sexual orientation. Although so gifted, each thing she created – and she was driven to create – was born out of anguish. Celia's fear of commitment also prevented her from finding a consistent or remunerative outlet for her talents. Finally she had become ill with severe Candida Albicans. (An imbalance in intestinal flora which, in extreme cases, affects many aspects of physical and mental functioning, causes food allergies and saps the vitality.)

Chakra work helped Celia considerably. She soon realised that her sacral chakra needed much help and healing. It was the source and focus of energies which found inadequate outlet, and had become both blocked *and* over-active. Her multi-faceted talents made it difficult for her to make choices. She was afraid of people, yet

needed them. Everything which could have been joy
turned into pain. She was seriously depressed.

Candida is an invasive condition and often, symbolically, can reflect a lack of inner balance in the masculine
and feminine energies.

Knowing that she could work meditatively with colours,
fragrances, visualizations and crystals to help her sacral
chakra gave Celia hope. In the past she had tried many
therapies but could not stay with any treatment long
enough for it to have effect. Beneath the depression lurked
anger and panic. Now she attuned almost daily to her
chakra, used her paints and pastels to draw its condition,
then visually flooded it with the amber and gold it needed.
The panic began to subside, she realised that healing takes
time and saw herself as being in a transition period. She no
longer labelled herself as 'hopeless and helpless'.
Rediscovering joy in her talents, she allowed them to
enrich her life. They were no longer a burden.

Soon Celia was able to commit herself to psycho-
therapy in order to deal with all the disempowerment
which came from her childhood years – classically for the
sacral chakra – from between the ages of three to eight
years old. She addressed the wider issues of her sexuality
and discovered a new joy in being a woman. Dietary
treatment for the Candida, which had never really been
effective before, now worked. Her vitality gradually
returned.

Celia maintains that the concentration on her chakra set
the other therapies free to work for her. She feels that her
healthier chakra has helped her to change old, ingrained
patterns more effectively. She trained as an art-therapist
and, until her marriage, worked with emotionally
disturbed children. She is now awaiting the birth of her
first child. Her home is full of sacral chakra colours and
has an ambience of warmth and welcome. Celia is happy
and fulfilled at last.

# THE KEY WORDS

## Security

The attributes of the sacral chakra lead out from those of the root, building on, and blending with them. When there has been 'good enough' nurturing and grounding for the root chakra, one of its gifts to the sacral is the quality of security. If the foundations of security have not been laid at the root chakra stage, then this will cause imbalance and blockages at the sacral chakra which will need to be cleared and healed.

## Sense of Others

This leads on naturally from security. Those who feed our security (or betray it) are the 'others' in our environment. The quality of the early sense of others affects our potential for mature relationships. Positive, loving recognition from those around the young child should be the essential basis for healthy individuality.

## Sexuality

This is to be interpreted in a wide sense. It relates directly to the act of sex, but also includes the acceptance of sexuality and what it means to be a man or woman in the present age and culture. What are the expectations, the norms, the challenges, the confrontations of gender and gender roles? Everything which concerns bodily structure, instinct and the autonomous aspects of sex belongs to the root chakra. *Consciousness* of sexuality and sexual choices are related to the sacral chakra.

There is common disillusionment with sex. Biblical teaching is often interpreted thus: 'Woman tempts man to carnal knowledge. After a short-lived honeymoon period her children are brought forth in pain and travail. The innocent have fallen, paradise is lost, woman is the temptress and sex is the reason.'

With those attitudes festering in our collective unconscious it is small wonder that our sex lives are so often complex and/or inhibited. The intricacies of family life and the struggles and responsibilities of survival have led to conflict between the sexes. The ideal of partnership and mutual support evaporates. It is little short of a miracle when the qualities of humour and joy, and the vision of a spiritual union, which *includes* sex, survive.

Many spiritual teachings see sex, and even procreation, as 'lower' activities to be transcended in the interests of spiritual strength. The confusion, if not the guilt, with which many spiritual seekers look on their sexuality is frightening.

It is not, however, only spiritual seekers who hold the view that human endeavour benefits from sexual abstinence. Dedicated athletes, great thinkers and creative people of all kinds eschew sexual activity before the big match, battle of wits or new project. The psychologist Freud gave us the concept of sexual 'sublimation'. It is often seen as a virtue to sublimate or transform sexual or 'primitive' urges into higher energy. We create an 'either/or' choice between sex and other fulfilling activities.

Apart from the Eastern teachings of 'Tantra' there is little guidance on sexual activity or union as a means to, and essential part of, spiritual experience. Few recognise the spiritual side of sexual energy. The beauty, wonder and level of spiritual communication in sex are only too frequently ignored.

Though Gildas gives his last incarnation as that of a monk in fourteenth century France, his views on sexuality are certainly not those of a monk. He links sex to creativity, co-creativity and empowerment. He encourages the view that enjoyment of sex and sensuality are not only part of the spiritual journey but enhance and energize it. Through sex we take part in the sacrament of creation. Sexual interaction of many kinds can enhance and fertilize all forms of creativity. Sexual exchange can release energy for work projects, artistic endeavours, decision making, sports prowess, book writing, or simply for openly creative living. In sex there can be a sharing of laughter, joy and delight in the life-force, as well as the ultimate communion and consummation of deep love.

The Transpersonal Psychologies recognize that anything which is suppressed, condemned or surrounded by guilt may become shadow material and gain autonomy. (See *Glossary* for information on 'Transpersonal Psychologies' and 'shadow material'.) It then rules us, in a negative way and is not a bright, honed tool to be used with skill and expertise. When sex becomes burdened with darkness and denial it breeds degradation, pornography and abuse. It becomes a source of fear and anxiety instead of delight.

When sexuality is seen as a life tool, then such issues as celibacy, sexual abstinence and continence also take on a different light. Gildas' teaching on sexuality is neither about undisciplined licentiousness nor sex as a required ingredient of the spiritual path. At certain times and according to choice, abstinence may be enlightening. Yet this should be a matter of free choice and acceptance. It should not come from a conviction that sex is intrinsically wrong and sinful. Abstinence can then enable observation of the body's natural signallings, rhythms and needs, without yielding to obsession by them or needing to punish the flesh for having desire in its juices. Working with the sacral chakra can lead to greater clarity about our sex lives.

## Creativity

A dictionary definition is: 'the state or quality of being creative. The ability to create.' The definition of 'create' is: 'to bring into being or form out of nothing; to bring into being by force of imagination; to make, produce or form; to design; to invest with a new form or character; to institute; to be the first to act; to make a fuss.'

As a teacher of young children, one of the most distressing things I found about large classes was the need to demand a high degree of conformity. In classes of over forty pupils it was easy for certain children to be labelled as 'deviant', 'demanding', 'attention-seeking' or 'nuisance'. They were almost invariably the most potentially creative. We live in a society which demands adaptation to a 'norm'. The gifted individual suffers and, like Celia, may not easily find effective help. Eccentricity is only marginally tolerated. There is an observable downward spiral of creativity → unusualness → non-conformity → non-acceptability → deviancy → delinquency, which is rarely imaginatively treated or healed. Such people all too often lead emotionally impoverished lives. They frequently end up in mental hospitals, prisons or other institutions.

Apart from the dictionary definition of 'create', I like to see it as the ability to bring two or more known factors together in order to form something new. For many people newness means change. The price we pay collectively for any over-emphasis on conformity is either resistance to change or addiction to change. Both positions mean that enlightened use of exploration, discovery and human potential is impossible and wise leaders do not emerge. In present times the collective sacral chakra needs much help and healing.

### Empowerment

This differs from power in that power is a *principle* and empowerment is the *process* of making use of that principle. Psychological empowerment is about having access to all our capabilities and potentials and not attending on some permission or approval from another or others in order to use them. The empowered person is creative and uses creativity to empower others.

This process must be strongly contrasted to that of 'giving away power'. When other people, parents or outer authorities are seen as manipulative, judgemental or limiting, it is possible that we are *giving* them this power. We may be *allowing* them to negatively influence our adult choices or to make unreasonable demands on our time and resources. If others are set on a pedestal and made into gurus or invincible leaders, our own roles are limited to those of disciples or followers. If the idol is discovered to have feet of clay, distress can be great and the recovery period long. The empowered person respects the authority, wisdom or expertise of another without self-belittlement and becomes more empowered by the contact. True teachers and leaders can empower others. They do not seek glamour or applause for its own sake.

## Co-creativity

This key word is about owning our part in anything which exists or happens in society. As a key word it is inseparable from empowerment. If we see authority as being totally to blame for anything and everything bad and totally to be praised for anything good, then we disempower ourselves. We deny the part we have in electing leaders and in forming the laws of society. Co-creativity is active. Being a victim is passive. Parents can do a great deal during the developmental stage for the sacral chakra to lay the foundations for co-creativity. Equally, parents and teachers are often disempowering to children, thus making co-creativity a difficult stance to attain.

Much religious dogma portrays God as anthropomorphic and over-authoritarian. This leads us to fear and to blame the creator and to see him/her as an over-responsible parent. When things go wrong in our world we may ask 'Is God dead?' – implying that were God alive we could be saved from ourselves. Rescued and forgiven, like the Prodigal son, we could be welcomed back as Innocents into the Garden of Eden.

God the parent certainly *needs* to die in order that we human beings can fully acknowledge our intrinsic potential to co-create a balanced and harmonious world. By drawing on the Infinite Source of Being we need to find the true formulae for survival and transcendence. Fully activating the sacral chakra can help in awakening the divine within each of us and in healing the schism between spirit and matter.

## Sincerity

This is a condition of freedom from pretence or deceit. 'The same in reality as in appearance or seeming or profession', is the Oxford Dictionary definition. When there is no fear of false authority or of persecution, it is easy to be sincere. This quality awakens naturally out of empowerment. Working with the chakras is serious and far-reaching. The sincere individual subjects the world to scrutiny under a bright and searching light. This is a clarifying and healing light, but often a confrontational one. Many interpersonal and intrapersonal values are challenged by it and may need to be renegotiated.

# THE DEVELOPMENTAL AGE

The functioning of the sacral chakra is strongly affected by the experiences we have between three/five to eight years old. As previously mentioned, the lower age is variable because there is a noticeably faster development in children now. Children tend to stay less time in the root chakra phase.

The developmental years relating to this chakra are those in which there is discovery and exploration of individuality. This phase can be both fascinating and exhausting for parents and teachers. The child needs boundaries but also flexibility. The warm and rich environment, so important to the root chakra, must continue. Pattern, repetition and routine help to maintain a framework of security. This framework nurtures the ability to see life as an exciting adventure of discovery.

At this age it would be unusual for a child to be aware of the deeper issues of sexuality, though there is a growing gender awareness and curiosity. Questions about the 'facts of life' are the norm and need to be answered as they arise. They should be neither circumvented nor answered in a detail for which the child may not be ready. When the question 'where did I come from?' is first asked some children receive an overwhelmingly detailed answer from a parent 'anxious to be open about these things'. The simple device of initially turning the question conversationally back to the child: 'What do you think?' may bring better insights into what is really being asked, so that the answer can be specific but not too detailed for the child's developing thought processes. Embarrassed avoidance may inhibit further inquiry, but so will too much inappropriate detail too soon. Careful handling of sensitive subjects with this age group lays good foundations for later attitudes in the handling of sexual expression and experience.

In these years children often have an experience of tenderly loving a friend of the opposite sex. It is important for parents and teachers to recognize how deep these feelings run. It is a mistake to ridicule or make fun of this early awakening.

The child already needs to be empowered. It is tempting to be over-protective, or over-authoritarian when the child's zest and energy for life is high. All parents have fears for their children's safety in one way or another. Boundaries, rhythms and routines are essential, but they must also be flexible if the sense of adventure and initiative is not to be repressed.

Adult empowerment happens more easily if early discipline has not been over-harsh or stifling. Unnecessary rebellion against authority, or obsessional self-control and ordering are polarities of behaviour which show that authority problems have not yet been dealt with. Such problems usually arise from unsatisfactory early experience. The empowered, creative adult can be happily conformist when necessary, while maintaining spontaneity and individuality of expression.

An over-judgemental or demanding environment affects the ability of children to be sincere, open and honest. Fear of retribution makes for deceitfulness. Wherever possible the child must be understood as an explorer of life and sympathetically helped to sort out mistakes which are made. It must also be noted that from this age onwards children demand absolute sincerity. Most parents can tell a 'was my face red' story about the confrontations which happen when 'little white lies' have been revealed in public.

Repressions, traumas and conflicts during this developmental stage have far-reaching effects and inflict wounds which take a long time to heal. The sacral chakra holds particularly vital energies for living. It is strongly linked to the throat chakra, which is the centre of expression. If the flow between these two centres is insufficient it is difficult to find a fulfilling role in life. Yet, because of its vitality, the sacral chakra has great healing potential both for itself and the whole being.

## THE COLOURS

These are colours of vitality. Orange in its more vivid forms is sometimes experienced as enervating or confrontational. In this case amber and gold should be used in visualizations and healing for the sacral chakra. When convalescing from illness, feeling tired or just needing an energy boost, visualizing orange light flowing into the sacral chakra is effective. A bowl of oranges in a room, or some orange or amber glass hanging in a window where sunlight can pass through it, can also be of help.

## THE ELEMENT

At the root chakra the element of earth gives fixity and stability. Water at the sacral brings a sense of movement. Water is linked to the moon. Symbolically it is often interpreted as governing the emotions. Inevitably it connects to time and tide, to fertility cycles, to the patterns of menstruation and ovulation in women and the production of seminal fluid in men. Earth and water define each other. Water courses cut their way even through the bed-rock of earth but the earth contains them. Without water, earth is infertile and inert. With it, earth becomes alive and productive. The element of water at the sacral chakra means that it is linked to bodily fluids such as the life force of blood, the hydration of the body and the fluid processes of cleansing and elimination.

## THE SENSE

Between three and eight years of age the growing child is introduced to wider varieties of foods and begins to build a spectrum of likes and dislikes. Yet the sense of taste is not only oral. It also relates to fashion, colour, architecture, design, entertainment and even political trends within society at any given time. The question linked to the sense, 'How do I taste the world, and how does the world taste me?' has wide implications.

Those who have difficulty in tasting food have been able to improve this sense by working with the sacral chakra.

## THE BODY

In constitution, the etheric body is a subtle 'double' of the physical body. It is the densest of the subtle bodies. Each of our vital organs has an etheric double interacting with the physical organs and helping to keep them healthy. Whether the etheric body receives subtle healing energies from a 'healer' or not, it has to repair itself before the physical organs can function normally once more. When any part of the physical body is amputated or removed, its etheric essence remains. The phantom limb is a medically accepted fact. The etheric body may be very traumatized and need intensive healing but it remains whole. Losing a physical organ does not mean losing its etheric counterpart. This is one of the reasons why the physical body is able to adapt and carry on functioning even when a relatively vital organ has to be removed. At death the etheric substance is an important agent in enabling the transition to the afterlife state. Some of the essences required can only be withdrawn if the whole physical body is dead. Serious complications have arisen because of organ transplants. Some parts of otherwise dead bodies are living on in other persons. The complete essence required for transition is then unavailable. This can result in 'waiting around' in a healing temple on the astral plane until the essence becomes available on the death of the organ recipient. Also, the person who loses an organ and receives a transplant, retains the etheric substance of the original organ. There is great difficulty in weaving the additional essence of a donated organ into the etheric structure of the recipient. It is small wonder that the greatest hazard of transplant surgery is the problem of rejection of the donated organ.

With the modern drugs of allopathic medicine we live under a delusion that healing has become a quickened process. Certainly many unpleasant symptoms can be eased but when symptoms disappear the journey of healing is not necessarily completed, especially for the etheric body. Recovery from illness needs time, rest and tender loving care, whether the symptoms have been miraculously 'cured' or not.

There is no denying that allopathy has produced many breakthroughs in healing but the subtle bodies have their own healing rhythm and may be adversely affected by one of the strong medicaments which remove physical symptoms. Resting when ill is sometimes seen as weak or undignified. Our present way of life can be over-demanding of our intricate constitution. Society often demands that we push ourselves too far.

## THE GLANDULAR CONNECTION

The lymphatics form a secondary transport system which helps to clear waste matter from the body. (Arteries, veins and blood are primary transport systems.) The lymphatics also help to restore plasma volume to the blood and to carry protein to the capillaries. Lymph nodes behind the knees, in the groin, under the arms and in the neck help to trap unwanted bacteria and other debris. They are part of the body's defence or warning system and may swell up when an infection is on the attack. When a hand is infected the underarm nodes swell into action. Those in the neck swell to fight throat infections. Where primary cancer is present and cells get into the lymphatic transport system, secondary growths will usually occur.

## THE FRAGRANCES

Musk and amber quieten the sacral centre while rosemary and rose geranium stimulate it. Musk oil is a plant product as is amber and these fragrances should not be confused with the animal extracts used in the perfume industry. Use the stimulating fragrances if you have a tendency to be rather passive, lacking in vitality, have difficulty in making choices or need more sexual vitality. Use the quietening fragrances if you are over-active, fear loss of control or find it difficult to 'play', relax or sleep.

## THE CRYSTALS AND GEMSTONES

Information on how to work with crystals and gemstones can be found on pages 174-7.

☆ *Amber* is not technically a crystal at all. It is the petrified resin of pine trees and exists in a number of different shades ranging from brown to yellow. It energizes, balances and heals. It lifts depression and aids dreams and creativity. It brings healing to the feminine reproductive organs and helps to regulate the menstrual cycle. This stone is also linked to the alter major and heart chakras.

☆ *Citrine* also comes in a variety of shades ranging from deep golden brown to stones which have a hint of lemony tinge in them but are otherwise clear. The orangey or amber citrines are most appropriate for this chakra. Since citrines are rarer than amethysts and yet in great demand, be sure when choosing a stone that you are not getting a heated amethyst posing as a citrine. Citrine heals wounded emotions and help emotional maturity. It aids the acceptance of sexuality and any work which needs to be done on sexual problems. It enhances the quality of generosity and encourages abundance.

☆ *Topaz* aids fertility. It attracts positive synchronicity and helps to promote inner peace.

☆ *Aventurine* helps in the release of blocked creativity and in activating the imagination.

☆ *Moonstone* is the stone of the moon goddess and protects all who travel on water. It can help us to see ourselves more as others see us. It enables greater conscious contact with our feelings. A feminine stone, it is useful to both men and women who are seeking to be more in touch with their feminine side. It aids dream memory. It helps in bringing projects to fruition and in clearing blocked creativity.

☆ *Jasper* is a stone of power and empowerment. The water element is often interpreted as being unstable and over-sensitive. Yet water can also be directed, active and full of power and energy. Jasper is the stone which reflects these latter qualities. At the sacral centre it is the foil for moonstone and amber and used together with these will help to balance the chakra.

## IN CONCLUSION

The sacral chakra is more complex than the root. It has more petals and more movement. Classical Indian philosophy gives it six petals. Its Sanskrit name is 'Svadhisthana' which means sweet or pleasurable. It is the second chakra in a team and the energies brought into being and affected by it are basic and powerful. The fully conscious development of any of the chakras is a life task. We come back again and again to some of the lessons associated with the sacral chakra especially in the emotional areas of life. The raw, gut-feeling emotions, the all-consuming passions of love, hate, anger or blind dedication to a cause belong to the water element in full power, majesty and flood. In this form the emotions tend to 'have us' rather than being fully available for more rational use and expression. Such emotions may fire creativity but can also be destructive. When gripped by something emotional in life we may say 'I am torn in two by it'. When the sacral chakra energy flows, split and conflict are easier to resolve. The flow to the heart chakra clears and raw emotion becomes tempered with wisdom and compassion.

## MEDITATIONS AND SUGGESTIONS FOR WORKING WITH YOUR SACRAL CHAKRA

### 1.   Contacting and Sensing the Sacral Chakra

Check the location of your sacral chakra on the diagram on page 5. Then use the root chakra sensing exercise on page 36, substituting 'sacral' for 'root' and follow this with the 'Images and Symbols' exercise on page 37.

## 2.   Guided Visual Meditation for the Sacral Chakra

Let your body be comfortable, poised and symmetrical.... Be in touch with the rhythm of your breathing and centre into your own inner space ... hear the sound of running water and find yourself walking through a wood in springtime, towards a stream ... the trees have young, delicate green leaves, through which the sun is shining and dappling the ground.... There is soft, moist leaf-mould underfoot ... there are scattered clumps of primroses ... birds are singing and are busy with their young ... the stream to which you have come is very clear.... It flows busily over a stony bed ... the ground is flat but the water flows down on to it from a higher source, beyond the trees and woodland, where there are rocks and less green growth.... You decide to follow the watercourse towards its source.... As you walk uphill, every so often you refresh yourself from the clear running water ... the channel through which it runs gets deeper but rockier as you go upwards ... after a while you are conscious of the noise of a waterfall coming from beyond some large rocks where the stream comes through a narrow opening.... You have to leave the stream and go around some rocks to the left ... as you swing back towards the stream, you find yourself in a rocky clearing ... Above you are great boulders and over them pours the gushing, foaming torrent of a waterfall.... The torrent falls into a natural, clear rocky pool, before forcing itself through the narrow gap in the rocks.... The sun is warm for springtime and high in the sky now, it falls on to the waterfall and the natural rock pool.... The light and the water form rainbows in the air but the pool itself is sparkling with golden and amber colour.... As you gaze into it your whole body seems to fill with warm and vital light.... Your sacral chakra in particular receives healing colour and energy ... fully refreshed, you dip your cupped hands into the pool and drink the water which, even as you drink, remains golden and vital ... there is a magical quality around and you are drawn to look into the water's depths.... Something is shining.... You know that it is a gift for you to take with you ... a talisman for your sacral chakra.... Reach in ... take it ... carry it with you as you return from this place, down beside the gurgling stream again, to the woodland where you began ... as you return, know that, once you have found a place in your inner space, you can always revisit it ... know that you can draw inner strength from the symbolic gift which you received at the mountain pool.... Return gently to the rhythm of your breathing ... to a full consciousness of your body ... to your contact with the ground ... to your every-day environment.... Visualize a cross of light in a circle of light over your sacral chakra and surround the whole of your aura and body with a cloak of white light with a hood.

## 3. Questions

Contemplate the questions 'How do I taste the world?' and 'How does the world taste me?'

## 4. Fragrances

Use the fragrances for this chakra, to activate it, calm it or balance it. See page 33 – 5 for directions and suggestions for the use of fragrances with the chakras.

## 5. Colours

Use the technique of 'breathing' into your sacral chakra, and 'feed' it with the colours given on page 40. Remember to visualize the colours as translucent. Close down the petals and visualize the cross or star in the circle of light to finish.

## 6. Getting in Touch with the Developmental Age and the Inner Child

(a) Think about your family life when you were between three to eight years old. Remember the creative, joyful times, the days which were full of colour and sunshine. Then

sense things which were less good, less flowing, less creative.
(b) Think about the sexual 'climate' in your home. What
attitudes were there to your developing sexuality and to sex
in general? Get an image for the sexual climate in your
family during your upbringing. Discuss this image with your
partner or with a friend.
(c) Think about the needs of your 'inner child'. Life is never
perfect and there will be things which were missing from
your early life. Something within you, which can be termed
the 'inner child' may still crave those things. Use a
photograph of yourself as a child and see if a part of you
needs reparenting, reassuring, or to be given permission to
carry the valuable activity of 'play' into adult life. (See
*Glossary* for a fuller definition of inner child.)

## 7.   The Prayer or Affirmation

Meditate and reflect on the words given on page 40.

## Chapter 5

# The Solar Plexus Chakra

**Location**   Just below the sternum, extending down to the navel (stem in corresponding position at the back).

**Key Words**   Logic, Reason, Opinion, Assimilation, Psychic-intuition

**Developmental Age**   8–12 years

**Colours**   Yellow, Gold, Rose

**Element**   Fire

**Sense**   Sight

**Body**   Astral

**Glandular Connections**   Adrenals

**Quietening Fragrances**   Vetivert, Rose

**Stimulating Fragrances**   Bergamot, Ylang-Ylang

**Crystals and Gemstones**   Yellow Citrine, Apatite, Calcite, Kunzite, Rose Quartz, Iron Pyrites (Fools' Gold), Topaz, Malachite

### Prayer or Affirmation

Through the gift of fire let reason, logic, opinion and assimilation become truly linked to inspiration that we are not bound within limitation and separation.

## Solar Plexus Case History

Peter was thirty-five years old when he first came for
advice about his spiritual life. He is very shy and sensitive.
At that time he was working in biological science. He was
becoming increasingly unhappy with the nature of some of
the research he was doing. It involved work for fertilizer
companies on how to get more crops, more often, from less
land and how to grow everything bigger and more perfect
looking.

Peter identified with the earth and felt that it was tired
and exploited. He knew that bigger and more perfect
looking crops tended to have less and less flavour. He was
bored, depressed and angry. He had explored several
forms of meditation, mostly from books. He became
frightened and wary after having to be treated
psychiatrically for a brief period when prolonged and
unsupervised meditation had led him into a near-
psychotic state. Yet he was still anxious to explore the
spiritual dimension and to bring greater meaning and
purpose into his life.

He said, 'If I felt more secure in myself, I could take
risks, but I am not. When I meditate now, I am afraid of
getting lost in another world. Some of my meditations are
frightening. I am having bad dreams.'

The risks which Peter wanted to take were connected
with his work, as well as with his spiritual life. He no
longer wanted to analyse, especially for commercial
purposes which were increasingly in conflict with his
awakening spiritual vision. He felt that he wanted to be a
healer or counsellor but did not know how to go about
making the necessary life-changes.

Many insecurity problems arise at the sacral centre, and
certainly Peter needed to work with the sacral/throat
chakra connection. His spiritual problems though, and his
fear of getting lost in other worlds, pointed to a lack of true
ego structure. Much of his uncertainty about change was

connected with being out of touch with his inner fire and motivation. He did not really know who he was and was too vulnerable for intensive spiritual practices.

The solar plexus covers a wide spectrum but, most important, is the centre of identity and selfhood. Although Peter needed careful and patient counselling to help him contact his true self, work with the solar plexus helped and supported this.

Beneath his depression lay anger. Strengthening the solar plexus with light, colour and healing helped him to overcome his fear and guilt and to release some of the fiery anger related to his upbringing and the limitations it had placed upon him. Releasing and having the anger accepted, enabled him to use this fiery energy to tackle the changes he wanted to make in his life. He became really excited about his potential as a healer. He was fortunate in being in a position where he could give up his current work, take time off to concentrate on his own growth and to embark on a course in homoeopathy.

He is now in his final year of training and looking forward to setting up as a homoeopathic practitioner. He is much more confident and, like many intrinsically shy people, has been able to cultivate his ability to listen to great advantage. His trained, analytical mind remembers subtle nuances, and draws clear conclusions. These attributes are now enhancing his gift for healing.

Peter still finds meditation difficult, but he has recognised that his love of music and nature brings him into a meditative state and refreshes him. He does not need intense spiritual disciplines. Although his fire energy is more readily accessible, Peter has learned to be more gentle with himself. His self-knowledge, gained through counselling and in his homoeopathy training, has helped him to be less afraid of his inner worlds. His dreams are becoming a source of guidance, rather than being threatening or fearful.

He is using some of his released fire energy to campaign

for causes like 'Friends of the Earth' and 'Greenpeace'. He has offered some of his experience and biological knowledge to these organizations, as a help in preparing factual literature.

## THE KEY WORDS

In order to understand the key words for the solar plexus it is necessary to consider the complexity of this centre. It is the centre of the lower will or ego, as well as being connected with the digestive system, the fire element, sight, vision and psychic energies.

### Logic, Reason and Opinion

Part of ego or personality formation is related to having a logical and reasonable approach to life and to being able to form and state personal opinions. An independent rationality is needed in order to make the decisions about life which allow us to reach our personal and full potential. When Peter came to me, he was conforming to an outer standard of success and ignoring the inner logic of his own wishes and aptitudes. Intellect and mind have an important relationship with the solar plexus. The processes of empowerment, referred to at the sacral centre, continue. In the search for individuality, it is necessary to challenge some of the expectations of society. It is not possible to form and affirm our personal belief systems without the qualities of logic, reason and opinion.

### Assimilation

The solar plexus is connected to the digestive system and to physical assimilation of food and nutrients. Assimilation is also to be understood here, in its widest sense, which includes the mental and psychological assimilation of knowledge and experience.

## Psychic-intuition

The word 'psychic' can be used in a number of different ways, and there is a considerable difference between the psychic and the spiritual. Psychological and esoteric languages sometimes use the same words to mean different things. Psychologically speaking, 'psychic' refers to that which is 'of the psyche' (see *Glossary*). It helps to describe the interacting personality and behaviour patterns which make each individual a unique and multi-faceted being.

In esoteric realms the word 'psychic' is used to denote a particular kind of sensitivity. The psychic individual may have premonitions, either in dreams or through 'hunches' and 'knowings'. Crystal ball gazers use the psychic faculty. Tarot card, palm and astrology readings are re-establishing themselves now as serious studies leading to valuable spiritual guidance. They are also practices which can be energized from a specifically psychic level. The psychic faculty itself is a valuable ingredient in intuition and spiritual practice. If it gets 'stuck', though, at the solar plexus level and isolated there, it becomes limited. Psychic guidance will tend to relate only to the material world, the future, our love lives, 'luck' and all the areas generally associated with 'fortune telling'. Only when integrated with the qualities of the heart and brow chakras does it become truly spiritual.

Psychic energy is responsible for phenomena such as telekinesis, spoon-bending, clock-stopping, poltergeist happenings and psychometry (the art of attuning to an object in order to find out something about its history or its previous owners). The police sometimes consult mediums with strong psychic faculties in order to find bodies, missing persons or objects.

The psychic world can be frightening but psychic energy is a necessary ingredient in the vision and power which enables us to see, define, implement and change our spiritual direction, where necessary.

## THE DEVELOPMENTAL AGE

The span of eight to twelve years marks big changes for the child. There is an emergence into greater independence of being, which can sometimes be difficult for parents to handle. It is important to realize that though the child is seeking and wanting more independence, serious difficulties can arise when children are pushed too hard or too soon into a world of adult responsibility where childish things are ridiculed. Many who come for counselling, particularly men, have suffered from being sent off to boarding school at this early age and often have great depths of unexpressed grief to explore. The child needs a subtle, growing independence with continued holding, softness and loving.

Children of this age range are demanding in a new way. Growing egos make themselves known and felt. Developing intellects are insatiable for facts and more facts about the world around and how it works. Information is devoured and digested with great rapidity and more is demanded. A rich and stimulating menu is required if intellectual deprivation and mental malnutrition are to be avoided.

During this period girls often overtake boys, particularly in physical development. Most twelve-year-old girls of today show some definite bodily signs of moving into puberty and womanhood. Certainly the twelve-year-old of either sex has moved a long way in the four years since the age of eight.

From this time onwards there are new difficulties and considerations for the parent. On the one hand there is the fascination of watching and helping young people to maturity, on the other hand there has to be great subtlety in managing the changing relationships and giving the right degree of freedom, combined with protection, which prevents inexperience from leading to disaster. The choices which the child is making, even at this comparatively early age, can have long-term implications, and great bitterness and resentment may ensue if there is not enough opportunity for choice. Peter said, 'My parents and teachers did all the choosing for me. I felt very unseen and unheard.'

### Rites of Passage

Progression through the chakras connects with the ancient, traditional honouring of rites of passage. The upper age of the solar plexus chakra may mark the onset of puberty. Societies, which we often regard as more primitive than ourselves, mark and celebrate this and other life changes more specifically than we do. Our rituals around the coming of age, marriage, birth and death are often uncertain. It can be healthy and reassuring to mark life-changes and to celebrate the moments when new responsibilities and privileges are taken on and old patterns left behind. Such recognitions help in the process of defining and redefining the changing relationship between parents and offspring. Celebration can be simple or lavish, but it is worth remembering that it can enhance family life and clarify issues which otherwise may remain undefined.

## THE COLOURS

Clear bright yellow is a mental colour. It is a helpful one to use when doing the sort of work or study which involves memorizing facts. Have yellow folders and accessories on your desk or in your study area. Try putting a yellowish bulb in your desk lamp.

For healing at the solar plexus, the gold and rose colours are best. Gold should be visualized like pure, gentle, golden sunlight. Actual sunlight on the solar plexus can help the metabolism, the eyesight and the overall sense of wellbeing in the physical body. The very word 'solar' links this centre to the sun and all which is light, fiery and conscious.

Rose brings the softness which the solar plexus also requires. It cannot be stressed often enough that the chakra system is interconnective and interdependent. It is important

not to create a completely rigid and over-specific compart-
mentalization. The primal instincts from the root chakra
lead into the gut-feeling emotions of the sacral. At the solar
plexus, as the ego-self develops, the raw emotions need
further assimilation. Rose pink can be a great help in making
this assimilation smooth and gentle.

## THE ELEMENT

Earth and water elements are considered to be mostly
feminine, receptive or yin in nature. Fire is more masculine,
active or yang.

Fire consumes, but also sets processes in motion, changes
things and enables assimilation. We may refer to ourselves as
burning with desire, passion or purpose. We say we are
'fired' by imagination or the spirit.

When the solar plexus is under-functioning we tend to get
stuck on an inappropriate treadmill and to be unable, as
Peter was, to see how to bring about creative change in our
lives. Vision, as well as action, can be blocked. An active fire
element, nourished by a well-functioning solar plexus,
brings enjoyment and passion into living.

An over-active solar plexus or fire element can make us
over fiery, dry-skinned, irritable, uncomfortable and prickly
to ourselves and others. In our bodies food may be burned up
too quickly and nutrients imperfectly absorbed.

## THE SENSE

Sight is stimulated by light and thus belongs to the fire
element. The word 'sight' at the solar plexus refers to
creative vision as well as to physical sight. A healthy solar
plexus enables us to plan our lives well and wisely, and to
know when the winds of change or chance are blowing in our
favour.

Visualizing the colour gold flooding the solar plexus will enhance both physical and metaphorical vision.

## THE BODY

The astral body consists of subtle flowing energies, and is yellow, gold, rose or a clear, slightly electric, silvery blue.

In near-death experiences people frequently report 'being' in another part of the room, watching what is happening to their physical body. Those who have survived serious accidents have reported watching their physical body being treated, while their consciousness or essence waits at a distance, away from the physical pain and distress. In these experiences the awareness is withdrawn to the astral body.

Many people become attracted to the spiritual path because of the possibility of learning 'astral travel'. In this altered state of consciousness, journeys through time and space become possible. Anyone who wants to work specifically with the astral body should consult a well-established esoteric school or find a trusted teacher.

The higher astral plane, described by esotericists and 'sensitives' is very beautiful. It has flowing landscapes and healing temples. It is the plane where there is a loving contact with guides, helpers and angelic beings.

Lower layers of the astral plane are less attractive. Thought forms and negative 'entities' populate these regions. Some of the experiences of bad drug 'trips' and schizophrenia can come from a vulnerability which precipitates an unwanted breakthrough into these realms. Some healers and psychic workers specialize in helping those who have come under these influences. See the *Glossary* for further information on 'astral'.

## THE GLANDULAR CONNECTION

There are two adrenal glands – the cortex and the medulla – which are in the abdomen, above the kidneys. Although anatomically linked, they serve different masters. The medulla is activated by nerve impulses, while the cortex is an endocrine gland, activated by blood-borne hormones, sent out by the pituitary.

The cortex hormones are essential to life. Cortisol is an energy generator, but is also in charge of energy storage and regulates the fire element in the body. Aldosterone prevents excessive loss of water through the kidneys and maintains the crucial bodily balance between sodium and potassium.

The medulla gives us the 'fight or flight' response by flooding the system with extra adrenalin when quick reactions are required.

When continually over-stressed, we use up adrenalin reserves faster than they can be replaced. We may then have a physical stress 'breakdown' and need a lot of rest and care in order to recuperate fully. Treating the solar plexus chakra helps to alleviate and prevent stress breakdowns.

## THE FRAGRANCES

Vetivert and rose quieten, while bergamot and ylang-ylang stimulate. (Bergamot is an ingredient in Earl Grey tea.) Use the quietening fragrances if you have digestive problems such as colitis or ulcers, if you have difficulty when mingling with crowds, travelling on the Underground etc and if you are at a transition point in your life. Use the stimulating fragrances if you have a slow metabolism, defective eyesight and fears about change.

## THE CRYSTALS AND GEMSTONES

Information on how to work with crystals and gemstones can be found on pages 174 – 7.

☆ *Citrine* has already been mentioned at the sacral centre. The brighter, clearer, yellower citrine is most useful to the solar plexus. It helps in cultivating clarity, warmth and the sense of self. It is also healing for digestive upsets.

☆ *Apatite* aids concentration and intellectual thought. It helps in the development of logical communication.

☆ *Calcite* comes in many colours. Orange, honey and yellow calcites aid psychic development. They are also helpful when studying. They help to connect the higher will to the lower will.

☆ *Kunzite* is usually pink. It aids self-discipline, self-respect, inner balance and the cultivation of gentle strength and compassion. It helps to strengthen non-judgemental but accurate self-observation.

☆ *Rose Quartz* helps to keep this chakra flexible. The solar plexus is a shock absorber. Under stress it gets brittle and rigid. If this happens rose quartz should be used.

☆ *Iron Pyrites* brings strength of purpose, helps all levels of assimilation and encourages the discovery of one's full potential.

☆ *Topaz* aids cheerfulness and humour. It helps to strengthen vision and purpose.

☆ *Malachite* aids psychic and spiritual abilities. It aids the remembrance of dreams. It is also healing for physical eyesight problems.

## IN CONCLUSION

Psychologically speaking the solar plexus is the ego centre, the place at which we confidently say 'I', and where we are in touch with our needs, desires and constructs about life and the world in which we live.

The oft-quoted spiritual injunction to 'lose the ego' is suspect and dangerous in its openness to misinterpretation. The ego is the identity. It must be strongly built before any wider explorations can take place with safety. Some psychotic conditions are linked to loss of identity. Eventually the ego may surrender with grace and joy to a sense of higher will and purpose. If it is a strong and well-honed tool, then it will carry the potential to be a better instrument for that higher will.

The Sanskrit word for the solar plexus is 'Manipura'. Classically it has ten petals.

## MEDITATIONS AND SUGGESTIONS FOR WORKING WITH YOUR SOLAR PLEXUS CHAKRA

### 1.   Contacting and Sensing Your Solar Plexus Chakra

Check the location of your solar plexus chakra on the diagram on page 5. Then use the sensing exercise on page 36. Then substituting 'solar plexus' where appropriate, follow this with the 'Images and Symbols' exercise on page 37.

### 2.   Guided Visual Meditation for the Solar Plexus Chakra

Begin by ensuring that you will be undisturbed, and then find a comfortable position in which to sit or lie . . . arrange your body symmetrically and let it relax . . . close your eyes and visualize the solar plexus colours . . . bright, clear yellow, soft golden yellow, and a gentle rosy pink. . . . As the colours surround you, they also warm you and your whole body feels more vital . . . imagine that you are sitting on a

hill top near the sea ... pine trees go right down almost to
the water's edge ... there is a bay, with a wide, sandy
beach.... The sun is warm and golden and the sea is many
colours of blue and bluey green.... It is clear and the waves
are gentle.... A little way out to sea is a small island ...
covered with pine trees, it seems to be almost perfectly
circular.... You make your way down to the beach ...
taking in the sounds, the smells and the beauty which
surround you.... Take off your shoes and explore the firm
sand at the water's edge, letting the gentle ebb and flow of the
tide wash over your feet and ankles.... You look again at
the island ... the sun shining on the sea is making a pathway
of light over the water towards the island ... and you decide
to follow it.... In the way which is possible in dreams and
meditations the pathway of light literally becomes a bridge
which you can walk over, to reach the island.... When you
arrive there, you follow a path through the pine trees.... It
seems to lead towards the centre of the island.... You are
wrapped in a deep sense of inner peace ... the ground you
are treading seems to be hallowed ground ... as you come to
the central point you see that there is a clearing which is
perfectly circular in shape.... At the centre of the clearing
there is an indentation which has been carefully and
beautifully lined with yellow, gold and pink crystals.... In
this crystalline basin burns a strong and steady flame ... as
you come nearer you know that you are approaching the very
centre of your being.... You find somewhere to sit so that
you can watch the reflection of the flame in the crystal
hollow ... you feel centred and at peace, in touch with your
basic identity ... totally accepted in every way.... You
know that this flame is *your* flame and that it has the power to
strengthen and validate your identity, your energy and your
sense of purpose in life.... Stay here in silent contemplation
for a while.... Then return to the edge of the island ...
back across the sunlit causeway ... to the beach ... back
into an awareness of your breath in your body, your contact
with the ground, your presence in your everyday world....

Remember that you can always return to the place of the flame, when you need inner strength and self-confirmation. . . . Put a cross of light in a circle of light over your solar plexus chakra and draw a cloak of white light with a hood around you . . . so taking the light into your life with you without being too vulnerable as you resume your normal tasks. . . .

### 3. Questions

Contemplate the questions: 'How do I see the world?' and 'How does the world see me?'

### 4. Fragrances

Use the fragrances for this chakra to activate it, calm it or balance it. (See pages 33 – 5 for directions and suggestions for working with fragrances.)

### 5. Colours

Use the technique of 'breathing' into your solar plexus chakra and 'feed' it with the colours given on page 59. Remember to visualize the colours as translucent. Close down the petals and visualize the cross or star in the circle of light to finish.

### 6. Getting in Touch with Other Factors

Consider your desires and your needs. What do you want from life? What do you need from life? Make clear distinctions between needs and desires. Some people's needs are other people's luxuries. Each person is an individual. Look at your desires without condemning them. Consider which you are making progress towards and which may be blocked. Consider whether you are still holding on to parental or authority messages about what is 'good' or 'right' for you. Try to know what you want, need or desire for yourself.

## 7.   Rites of Passage

Consider the time of your puberty, and whether it was satisfactorily marked for you as a rite of passage. Is there anything in your life right now which you would like to celebrate? If so, think of a private or more public celebration and arrange it.

## 8.   The Prayer or Affirmation

Meditate and reflect on the words given on page 59.

# Chapter 6
# The Heart Chakra

**Location**  On the same level as the physical heart but in the centre of the body (stem at back).

**Key Words**  Compassion, Feeling, Tenderness, Love of God, Love of Others, Detachment

**Developmental Age**  12–15 years

**Colours**  Spring Green, Rose, Rose Amethyst

**Element**  Air

**Sense**  Touch

**Body**  Feeling

**Glandular Connection**  Thymus

**Quietening Fragrances**  Sandalwood, Rose

**Stimulating Fragrances**  Pine, Honeysuckle

**Crystals and Gemstones**  Emerald, Green Calcite, Amber, Azurite, Chrysoberyl, Jade, Rose and Watermelon Tourmalines

### Prayer or Affirmation

In the golden centre of the rose of the heart may tender compassion be linked to unconditional love. May true detachment enable growth and continuity. Through the understanding of birth within death and death within birth may there be transformation.

## Heart Chakra Case History

Imogen is a healer. Her clients speak highly of her healing talents, her caring and her dedication. She has been described as 'all open-heartedness and love'.

Six months ago Imogen went for a medical check-up, due to her increasing tiredness. She was found to be suffering from stress and was warned about a weakness in her heart.

This story is all too familiar among healers and carers. Carers tend to go around with wide open hearts looking after everyone except themselves. It can be very difficult to shed the troubles other people bring to you. When Imogen took the 'holiday' which many of her friends had been urging her to take, she went to the seaside with her daughter and family, which involved spending a lot of time dealing with her mentally handicapped grandson, so as to give her daughter a rest. 'It was very nice self-catering accommodation,' she said, 'near the beach, and Jimmy had a really happy time.' It did not take much reading between the lines to realize that Imogen had spent her whole time shopping, cooking and baby-sitting. Of course, she had loved every minute of it. She is justifiably proud of her family and they love and appreciate her but it was by no means the restful, lazy holiday which Imogen needed. It was shortly after this that she realized her tiredness was abnormal and that she had other symptoms which needed a check-up.

The pattern illustrated by Imogen's case is that of an over-active, and wide-open heart chakra. All her love and caring was flowing out towards others. The chakra, as well as the physical heart, was exhausted. It had lost flexibility. Imogen was rather taken aback when she came to me for help and I suggested that the first thing she needed to learn was to close the petals of her heart chakra.

I did not mean that she should cease to be the caring, demonstrative person she is. Just that sometimes, when she is alone and certainly before she sleeps, she should consciously put herself in a suitable frame of mind to replenish her own energies. Imogen realized that she could not carry on as she was. Being tired and ill meant that she was being prevented from helping others. It was very difficult for her to accept help, healing and concern, but we persevered. Spiritual healing helped her heart chakra to be more flexible. She also worked, in a relaxed and meditative state, to visualize the petals of her heart chakra opening and closing, opening and closing. Thus the flexibility increased and Imogen realized that she felt much better and less vulnerable when the petals of her heart chakra stayed loosely closed. In this way she maintained her own sense of wellbeing without feeling that she was shutting down completely to heart contact with others.

When I tuned in to the colours in her heart chakra, they were very pale and lacked vitality. Colour healing helped, but Imogen's own visualization of colour for her chakra was also important.

Gradually Imogen learned to take time to indulge herself and to relax completely. She did all the things she was advised to do medically and combined these with receiving healing and focusing on self-healing techniques. She is doing well, but it takes time to change deeply formed patterns of behaviour.

In a psychological sense Imogen was over-compensating. Her adolescence had been difficult. When she was fourteen years old her mother died of cancer. It was a long illness. Imogen, as the eldest of three children, experienced early grief and had to carry great responsibility. Such experience could have caused her to close her heart chakra down and become too self-contained and distant. Indeed she found the sense of belonging and family which she had missed in caring for others. In so doing she had forgotten how to 'play' and had to learn again.

# THE KEY WORDS

## Compassion

The roots of the word mean 'with passion', implying a feeling of identification with a person, cause, or life dilemma. Compassion brings non-judgemental understanding. From the Red Indian culture comes the saying: 'Judge no one, until you have walked at least a mile in their moccasins.' This reflects the true meaning of compassion.

## Feeling

In the heart chakra, basic emotions are converted into true feeling. There is a progression from the gut-level emotions at the sacral centre, through the awareness of self in the solar plexus to the quality of feeling, tempered with wisdom, which comes from a developed heart chakra. The heart-centred individual brings a feeling quality to life without being governed and driven by raw emotions. It is possible to have, acknowledge and use feeling without it controlling our lives in a way which evades rationality and responsibility. The emotions can be harnessed without being denied. Their energy can be used advisedly, enhancing self-respect and empowerment.

## Tenderness

Tenderness is here understood not only in its active state, of being tender towards others, but as a quality of being. When we exhibit our greatest strengths we are, at the same time, tender and vulnerable. As the heart opens we reveal and declare ourselves to the world. We put ourselves 'on the line'. It is only when we are prepared to be vulnerable and tender in this way that we can give tenderness, true feeling and compassion to others.

## Love of God

Some people may prefer another word than 'God' here. It is used to refer to the source of all being and not in an unconsciously discriminatory manner. The heart energy inspires a love of the mysteries of life and moves us to more than an intellectual or philosophical basis for living. Those who live from the heart have an intrinsic – but not naive – faith in a positive pattern and meaning which underlie our existence and govern our potential.

### Love of Others

This speaks for itself. Imogen, with her open heart, has a great love of others. Healthy love of self is also necessary, but far more difficult. The developed heart chakra enables a balanced two-way flow.

### Detachment

This does not mean cold or uncaring withdrawal, but the lack of this quality caused Imogen to end up in difficulties. Helpers need to achieve the discipline which enables them to see a situation with the detachment which brings clarity leading to dispassionate appraisal of problems. In this sense, detachment becomes the midwife who brings love and wisdom to birth.

## THE DEVELOPMENTAL AGE

Young people of twelve to fifteen years old are often tender and vulnerable. Responsive to the world, they are passionate about causes, daringly open to experience, engaged in the pangs and intensities of first love, involved in keeping journals, and inspired to write poetry.

This age group continues to need support and yet sufficient freedom to explore. Issues of trust between parents and children often become fraught. The honouring of a girl as a developing young woman by her father and of the boy emerging into manhood by his mother, present challenges which some parents find difficult to meet. If the young person is to develop maturity and self-assurance as an adult, permission and recognition must be given by the parent of the opposite sex from puberty onwards. Many single parents find this time very difficult indeed. If the other parent is absent an understanding uncle or aunt can often help by stepping into the breach. Grandparents, too, can be great allies. Failure to convey these important messages contribute to the child/woman or the Peter Pan/man syndromes, where development into true maturity is arrested.

Because many parents are aware that their children need empathy, loving counsel and permission, some young people have been known to comment that 'there is nothing to kick against'. It seems that parents have to resign themselves to the fact that they can never be perfect. Adolescence carries an intrinsic need for rebellion and the young person has to find something on which to focus the energy of discontent. The only thing to do is to recognize this stage as healthy. Parents should not be ashamed of their own values or of stating them, but still must make time to explain lucidly why they have the beliefs and standards they do. Having a child who is throwing out challenges brings an opportunity for greater consciousness of personal integrity and the basis on which rules and guidelines are formulated. Openness to change is also a heart quality.

At a physical level, trauma connected with this developmental stage can trigger asthmatic and allergic conditions. Some asthmas and eczemas exist from birth onwards and can be caused by over-anxious mothering. The mother may have a wounded heart chakra herself, which affects the child's early response to life.

## THE COLOURS

Spring green is the colour of young beech leaves in early spring. Rose is a gentle rose pink; rose quartz crystals give the right depth and quality for this heart colour. Rose amethyst is a deeper rose colour, with a touch of mauve or amethyst in it, making it a bluer pink.

Spring green heals the pain which come from being over-vulnerable to life and helps to open the heart when it has 'hardened' as a result of opposition or devastating emotional experiences.

Rose brings warmth and softness. It is comforting to the bereaved. Rose amethyst is strengthening to the heart after debilitating illnesses or in stress conditions. It balances blood pressure.

## THE ELEMENT

Air as the element for the heart chakra challenges those ideas about the heart, which link it mainly and symbolically, to romantic love. Air is a masculine/active/yang element. These air borne qualities give the heart its key word of detachment and demand a differentiation between romantic feeling, emotional feeling and the clear evaluatory feeling which is an ingredient of wisdom.

Our physical bodies need each element, but death comes most quickly when we are deprived of air. We contain air. We exist in air. We are touched by it. It gives us the important spaces between things which enable them to be defined. The ultimate physical closeness to another person is when we share the very breath they breathe. If we have seen the heart as over-romantic and the air element as too cold, distant and intellectual, then there should be a reconsideration in order to come to a true understanding of the heart chakra.

## THE SENSE

Being touched and allowing ourselves to be touched by others is important. Children deprived of closeness and touch suffer in their development. Yet touch is also to be understood as tenderness and vulnerability. We are touched by feelings and emotions. Situations touch, or move us to compassion. Being touched in this way inspires the actions which bring humane changes in society.

## THE BODY

When awareness is projected into the feeling body, people and objects are experienced in a special way. We enter a state of contemplation, which is a deep level of meditation and in which there is full identification with other people, trees, rocks, plants, crystals or animals. We experience them from within and sense the nature of their being, their rhythms and life-cycles. It is the feeling body which enables the ultimate mystical experience of total oneness described by contemplatives and poets. Those earth shattering, totally satisfying sexual orgasms are its product too.

This body has a vital, less fluid texture than the preceding astral body. The use of the heart colours in the environment, or placed around you when you meditate will aid its development.

## THE GLANDULAR CONNECTION

The secrets of the functioning of some glands in the body remain something of a mystery, even to modern medical science. The thymus is one of these. It is part of the lymphatic system, situated directly below the thyroid and parathyroid glands. It secretes a hormone known as thymic humoral factor, and between the ages of twelve to fifteen years begins to reduce in size. It is thought to have a connection with growth and with the progression from childhood to adulthood.

# THE FRAGRANCES

Sandalwood and rose quieten the heart chakra, while pine and honeysuckle stimulate it. Imogen uses the quietening fragrances as perfume, bath oil and in the environment as a help in her healing process. People who find the expression of feelings difficult or who are hesitant about touching and being touched, benefit from pine and/or honeysuckle.

# THE CRYSTALS AND GEMSTONES

Information on how to work with crystals and gemstones can be found on pages 174 – 7.

☆ *Emerald* helps to develop loyalty, trust, romantic love and spiritual love. It aids the balancing of heart and mind and the development of wisdom.

☆ *Green Calcite* heals all the subtle bodies, but particularly the feeling body. It also helps communication between head and heart. It brings strength during periods of change or transition. It helps to heal the wounds of the heart and to develop positive tenderness.

☆ *Amber* in all its shades resonates with the heart chakra. It is purifying and helps to develop balance and love.

☆ *Azurite* aids compassion. It is linked to the air element and is helpful in healing allergies and asthma.

☆ *Chrysoberyl* has many different colours and forms. (Emerald is one of them.) These lovely, but comparatively rare and expensive stones attract kindness and generosity. They aid forgiveness and revitalize all energies. They are sometimes called the 'stone of perpetual youth'.

☆ *Jade* Green or white jade helps to regulate the heart beat and increase vitality, longevity and life-force. It also helps in the cultivation of serenity, wisdom, harmony and perspective.

☆ *Tourmaline* appears in a wide range of colours, but the rose or watermelon varieties are most helpful to the heart chakra. Tourmalines aid tolerance, flexibility, compassion and transformation. They promote harmony, and help in the development of fine discrimination without judgementalism. They are helpful when the heart chakra may have closed down or become blocked through trauma, loss or bereavement.

## IN CONCLUSION

The solar plexus is the centre of our ego-structure, but the heart is the central chakra. It is a meeting place for the energies which feed down into it from the upper chakras and those which feed upwards from below.

The pulsation of the healthy heart chakra is the same as the pulse of a steady heartbeat. This pulse rhythm is universal and when the chakra is balanced we are at peace with others and the environment.

The Sanskrit name for the heart is 'Anahata'. Classically it has twelve petals.

## MEDITATIONS AND SUGGESTIONS FOR WORKING WITH YOUR HEART CHAKRA

### 1. Contacting and Sensing Your Heart Chakra

Check the location of your heart chakra on the diagram on page 5. Then use the sensing exercise on page 36, substituting 'heart' where appropriate. Follow this with the 'Images and Symbols' exercise on page 37.

## 2.  Guided Visual Meditation for the Heart Chakra

Sit or lie comfortably, with your body symmetrically arranged, balanced and relaxed . . . close your eyes and be in touch with the rhythm of your breathing . . . bring the breath rhythm into your heart chakra – in the centre of your body, on a level with your physical heart – sense your heart chakra like a rose which is about to open . . . it has a delicate fragrance . . . its outer petals are spring green while within there is a promise of a delicate rosy pink . . . the colours are translucent, ethereal and yet the rose itself has substance . . . with each in-breath and out-breath the petals unfold, releasing more and more of its fragrance . . . the heart centre colours surround you . . . as the centre of the rose reveals itself, you see that the base of each petal has a delicate amethyst light and tinge . . . your heart centre is pulsating and turning. . . . As its movement finds a steady rhythm and the colour and light increase, reflect on people in your life who need healing . . . any situations which need deeper understanding. . . . Do not allow yourself to pursue reasons, arguments or outcomes, just hold each person or situation in the light and fragrance of your heart centre, breathing steadily . . . you will gradually become aware of a constant pulsing rhythm in your heart centre . . . a rhythm which links with the central rhythm of the universe . . . with the rhythms of earth and the sea . . . with currents of air . . . and with the flicker of flames in a gentle, warming fire. . . . You begin to feel healed and vitalized too. . . . Experience this rhythm and healing for as long as you wish. . . . When you are ready to return, let the petals of your heart chakra gradually begin to fold in again . . . let them just relax. . . . If the centre was rather tightly closed into its bud when you began this meditation, try to let it be more loosely closed and relaxed now. . . . If you found it rather open, then try to finish with a sense of its being more resilient.... See spring green light all around and over the flower of your heart chakra ... then, through the rhythm of your breath, return to an awareness of your body, your contact with the ground and your normal everyday surroundings ... put a cross of white light in a circle of white light over your heart chakra and a cloak of white light with a hood right around you.... Feel your feet firmly in contact with the ground before you resume your normal tasks.

## 3. Questions

Contemplate the questions 'How do I touch the world?' and 'How does the world touch me?'

## 4. Fragrances

Use the fragrances for this chakra to activate it, calm it, or balance it. (See pages 33 – 5 for directions and suggestions for working with fragrances.)

## 5. Colours

Use the technique of 'breathing' into your heart chakra and 'feed' it with the colours given on page 74. Remember to visualize translucent colours. Close down the petals and visualize the cross or star of light in the circle of light to finish.

## 6. Getting in Touch with the Developmental Age

Reflect on the period of your life between twelve and fifteen years of age. What was your relationship like with parents and teachers? How romantic were you? What were your ideals, hopes and fears? How far have these: (a) changed? (b) been fulfilled? (c) been frustrated?

## 7. Masculine and Feminine Principles

Reflect on the active/masculine/yang and the receptive/feminine/yin aspects of your nature. The masculine principal has been defined as 'focused attention', and the feminine as 'diffuse awareness'. How easy/difficult is it for you to consider both **principles**, without getting confused about the traditional role models given to men and women by society? How easy/uneasy are you in the gender which is yours for this incarnation? How do these issues affect balance and harmony in your life and relationships?

## 8.    The Prayer or Affirmation

Meditate and reflect on the words given on page 74.

## Chapter 7

# The Throat Chakra

**Location** The neck (petals at the front, stem at the back).

**Key Words** Expression, Responsibility, Communication, Universal Truth

**Developmental Age** 15–21 years

**Colours** Blue, Silver, Turquoise

**Element** Ether/Akasha

**Sense** Hearing

**Body** Mental

**Glandular Connections** Thyroid and Parathyroids

**Quietening Fragrances** Lavender, Hyacinth

**Stimulating Fragrances** Patchouli, White Musk

**Crystals and Gemstones** Lapis Lazuli, Aquamarine, Sodalite, Turquoise, Sapphire

### Prayer or Affirmation

Help us to develop responsibility. May universal truth impregnate causal action so that the voice of humanity may find true harmony with the voice of the earth.

### Throat Chakra Case History

The first intimation that Frank's problems were connected with his throat chakra was revealed as soon as he spoke. He was a tall, well-built, handsome man in his early fifties. His voice was soft, rather high-pitched and monotonous. He frequently 'cleared' his throat. It was obvious that Frank found it difficult to express himself but his story gradually unfolded.

At eighteen years of age, not long before compulsory enlistment ended, he had been 'called up' for National Service. He had dreamed of becoming a vet and was hoping to join the Veterinary Corps but, in true army tradition, was posted to a tank regiment. Something in him died and when he left the army he could not find the drive to resume his interrupted studies. He entered the civil service and took up an administrative position. He was stifled by city and office life and totally unfulfilled. He regarded himself as a dull, uninteresting person with little or nothing to offer. Even attempts at having a relationship had been abandoned. Frank had his own reasonably comfortable flat conveniently near to his mother. His father had died early, from a heart attack. His mother had been very independent at first, but was now becoming increasingly crippled with arthritis and asthma. She needed a lot of help and support from Frank with the organization of her life. She had recently asked him to move in with her. This request had made Frank take a long look at himself again. He found the prospect of his boring job, combined with being a live-in help to his mother, appalling.

His life was dull, but at least he had freedom. He was widely read and had a passion for music and opera. He had sophisticated sound equipment in his flat and spent much of his leisure time listening to and studying the famous works. Occasionally he would go, alone, to an opera. His few experiences of travel had always been linked to opportunities to hear famous orchestras or visit the big-name opera houses. If he went to live with his mother, he would probably have to forfeit even these modest enjoyments.

Frank came to me, driven by despair. Healing and counselling were alien territories for him but he was ready to try anything. I gave him healing for his throat chakra and asked him to listen every day to a relaxation tape which incorporated visualization for this chakra. In fortnightly healing sessions, I encouraged him to talk about the visions and aspirations of his youth. He needed to grieve over what had been lost. I took advantage of his desperation to persuade him to go to some voice workshops. Gradually his throat chakra, which had been tight, constricted and too bright in its colours, began to relax and balance. Now, Frank smiled more often, his voice changed and he had a new-found vitality.

Quite shyly, at the start of one session, Frank told me that he had joined an introduction agency. I admired his courage and, over the coming months, his perseverance. At last his story had an almost fairytale ending. He met a woman of his own age, also an opera lover, who was widowed and living in quite a large house, with land, in the country. Eventually they married. Today Frank commutes to work. As soon as possible he is going to take early retirement and he and his wife hope to open a boarding kennels and cattery. Frank still visits his mother regularly. She gets on well with his new wife who has found a reliable help for her. Seeing Frank happily settled has enabled her to assert some of her old independence. When the time comes, she will accept Frank's financial assistance and probably move into a nursing home near him and his wife. Life and its possibilities has expanded for all three of them. Frank is finding compensation for his lost earlier opportunities. He is grateful for the healing I gave him but still rather suspicious about the spiritual path. Yet the throat chakra has a dual function and its activation and healing will probably lead him, in time, to seek a deeper understanding of the mysteries of life.

## THE DUAL FUNCTION OF THE THROAT CHAKRA

The heart chakra is a meeting and blending place for the energies which flow down from the crown and up from the root, while the throat chakra is a gateway. The sevenfold chakra system is sub-divided into two interacting groups and the throat is a member of both. As one of the five lower chakras it is related to an element, a developmental age and a sense. As the first of three upper chakras it is concerned with transpersonal expression and the connections to higher-self, spirit and soul.

When the three upper chakras are open and developed, an increasing sense of the need to serve humanity, without living in isolation, is often experienced. Service to the collective becomes a necessary and intrinsic part of self-growth and awareness.

## THE KEY WORDS

These have a dual level of meaning in accordance with the dual functioning of the throat chakra.

### Expression

At the first level expression means seeking fulfilment through having an outlet for all one's particular and special talents or abilities. One needs to find one's voice and to be heard, literally and metaphorically.

At the higher level, expression is concerned with connection to one's spiritual qualities. There is a need to be uncompromisingly true to self, to the extent of questioning or requestioning all previous expectations of self and others.

## Responsibility

This is first of all about taking charge of one's life, becoming adult, going through the rite of passage of 'coming of age' and all the issues connected with these.

At the second stage it is concerned with responding to, and interpreting the requirements of, a Divine or Higher purpose. Vocation is a 'calling' which is 'heard'. Responsibility at this second level is about hearing that calling and responding to it with conviction.

## Communication

Life itself is dependent upon communication. Every moment of every day and night, highly complex communications are taking place in our physical bodies. This is so from the moment of conception to the moment of death. Each body part is dependent upon another, though we may only become aware of the existence of this interdependent communication system within us when there is a minor or major breakdown, for example, when we eat something which causes our digestive system to grumble or we catch an acute dose of flu and discover that our limbs will not do what we require of them. In times of health and wellbeing the signallings of this miraculous and finely tuned inner communication system remain unconscious and are taken for granted. Working with the throat chakra can help in the important task of listening to our bodies and becoming more attuned to, and therefore more responsible for regulating, our health patterns.

We use communication to express ourselves in the world and to enable life, in another sense, to move on. It is required for the expression of ideas, the exchange of information and for building up the data which helps us in the endeavour to understand the world in which we live. The sophisticated communication systems of our present times mean that we are growing more aware of the lives and predicaments of our fellow human beings all over the world. The demand for mediumship or 'channelling' which expands our communication into other realms is very strong at this time too.

In her book about chakras (see *Bibliography*) Judith Anodea describes the creative function of communication thus: 'Communication creates the future. If I say to you, "Bring me a glass of water," I am creating a future for myself which contains a glass of water in my hand. If I say, "Go away, leave me alone," I am creating a future without you. From presidential speeches and corporate board meetings to friendly discussions or marital fights, communication is creating the world at each and every moment. The Hindus believe that all is a matter of sound. Our own sounds create the shape of things around us at each vibration.'

Frank's voice had been constrained and he had lost the vision of a different quality of life. Many factors were involved so it is too simplistic to say that when Frank's voice changed, his life changed. Yet there is a definite connection between the sounds we make and the sort of lives we live.

Understanding the second level here can be facilitated by meditating on the opening verses of St John's gospel, 'In the beginning was the Word, and the Word was with God and the Word was God. The same was in the beginning with God. All things were made by him; and without him was not anything made that was made. In him was life; and the life was the light of men. And the light shineth in darkness and the darkness comprehended it not.' Some scientists are beginning to believe that sound is the basic pattern which enabled the universe to come into being. If time proves this to be so, then these verses can be seen as an inspirational statement about the laws of physics. It is more usual to understand them philosophically, thus: through concept, given form by language and verbally communicated, creation happens. So awareness of the throat chakra is vital if we are to realize our full potential.

## Universal Truth

At the first level this key word connects the throat chakra to law and order. The normally functioning human being needs to have a sense of moral rightness. Collectively formed laws derive partly from this drive and its recognition. Individually, we strive for integrity and function best when we refuse to make negative compromises.

At the second level, universal truth is concerned with a search for understanding of 'Divine law' or the archetypes of higher qualities. It is the search in which the questions 'What is beauty/peace/justice/wisdom?' are pertinent and challenging.

# THE DEVELOPMENTAL AGE

In the sevenfold system, this is the final chakra to be connected with a specific developmental age and a sense. The higher and new chakras are more general in their application with the exception of the base, which affects the gestation period.

Between fifteen to twenty-one years there are study and exam pressures on young people. There is preparation for 'coming of age', career choices, and escaping the parental sway. The influence of the key words can clearly be seen. Young people making career choices often feel a sense of vocation. They know beyond all doubt that they are 'called' to express something specific or have a special mission. Just as often they are confused. The present state of unemployment does not alleviate these problems.

Parents hope that their children will 'do well' and in this wish, tend to reflect the prevailing society trends of what is most 'acceptable' or 'successful'. Many young people go along with the traditional thought. They may genuinely want to fit into society's current dictation of success standards for the whole of their lives and will be happy and fulfilled in doing so. Others will rebel at being pushed into a mould or 'groomed for success'. It can be difficult for all concerned when the 'high flyer' with top performance in all exams and a seemingly brilliant conventional career ahead, decides to 'opt out'. Yet many who make far-reaching choices too soon or who fulfil the expectations of others rather than themselves will go through a particularly uncomfortable mid-life crisis. In the spiral of development the second level of the throat chakra has to manifest. Transpersonal psychologies have long encompassed a crucial life-phase which occurs around the age of forty-two years – twice twenty-one – when drastic life and career changes may be made. Frank had 'soldiered on' for rather longer than usual and as a result, the changes he *could* make were, at least outwardly, more limited.

## THE COLOURS

The whole range of blues, from palest to darkest, affect the throat chakra. The most common one recommended for healing use is deep lapis lazuli blue. Turquoises and aquamarines are particularly valuable in strengthening the ability to communicate with large groups or audiences. Career teachers, writers and those in the media can benefit from wearing and meditating on these hues. Silver is strengthening to the throat chakra and should always be visualized when throat infections occur. All these colours also affect the thyroids and parathyroids.

## THE ELEMENT

Ether, as an element, is not the same as the chemical solvent and anaesthetic. It is the element of the etheric body and the etheric plane, although these are mainly accessible via the sacral chakra, which has very strong connections to the throat. The etheric plane is the closest one to the physical or material plane. It is the first plane of subtle substance. We do not know what constitutes subtle substance, though many scientists believe in its existence and have described it as 'space' or the area in which electro-magnetic waves can be transmitted. Many discarnate guides, including Gildas, describe it as the layer, or other field of consciousness, from which the wonders of sound and colour originate. The Sanskrit word for ether is 'akasha'. In esoteric language the 'akashic records' are the imprint of all humankind's individual and collective experience. Nothing is lost, all is stored. Jung explored this belief psychologically in his writings about the 'collective unconscious'.

At the throat chakra ether can be seen not only as that element which records everything which has happened, but also as the blueprint. Thoughts, creative imaginings, concepts, are held here as part of their journey into the level which we know, in the body, as solid – the earthly 'reality'.

## THE SENSE

With sound frequencies as part of the etheric plane, and conceptualization and naming as important features at the throat chakra, hearing is the obvious connected sense. It is connected not only to listening, but to speaking, to being heard and to the quality of the voice.

## THE BODY

The mental body has a fluid texture and often reflects the throat chakra colours of blue, silver and turquoise. As its name implies, it is partly connected to intellect and abstract thought, to the world of ideas, conceptual blueprints and archetypes. (See *Glossary*.) It links us to the unseen patterns, subtle nuances and barely heard sounds which are aspects of complex communication. It enables divine principles to be apprehended, named and implemented.

Discarnate guides sometimes use the mental plane as their avenue of communication. The receiving medium then has difficulty in explaining how the communication happens. The mental bodies of guide and medium meet, and concepts or symbols which still require description are received. When the discarnate communicator and medium also engage their heart and brow chakras, more direct verbal communication with greater precision as to words and language style is possible.

## THE GLANDULAR CONNECTIONS

The thyroid and parathyroid glands are part of the endocrine system and secrete their vital hormones according to the signals from the pituitary which might be called the 'conductor of the endocrine orchestra'. The thyroid and parathyroids are situated in the neck. Thyroxine affects metabolism, bodily heat control and many aspects of growth. If there is too much the body will go into over-active stress; too little and everything becomes too slow. Children without properly functioning thyroid glands develop cretinism because this hormone is essential to the development of the intellect.

The parathyroids are contained within the thyroid itself and secrete a hormone which maintains the correct levels of calcium in the blood. Muscle activity of all kinds, including heart function, depends on correct levels of calcium in the blood plasma.

## THE FRAGRANCES

Lavender and hyacinth quieten this chakra while patchouli and white musk stimulate it. People who have tense, high pitched, nervous voices usually need the quietening fragrances, as do those who are over-talkative or over anxious about finding the right work. Those who speak too softly or hardly at all, who are obviously under-achieving in their work and are unfulfilled but confused as to what to do about it, need the stimulating fragrances.

## THE CRYSTALS

*Lapis Lazuli* aids expression of all kinds. It is helpful in healing deafness. It is a good crystal to have if you want to develop a musical talent or the art of colour co-ordination.

☆ *Aquamarine* assists in the easing of fears and phobias. It is an excellent stone for writers, journalists, and people who work in the media, as it aids positive communication with large audiences.

☆ *Sodalite* is often mistaken for lapis lazuli. It has a similar depth of blue colour but lacks the gold spots which distinguish lapis. It is excellent for healing all throat conditions and the thyroid gland.

☆ *Turquoise* is a favourite stone of the American Indians. It aids in the search for true purpose by helping attunement to the higher self or 'great spirit'. It provides clarity in all forms of communication.

☆ *Sapphire* is said to enable communication with beings from other planets. It strengthens the throat chakra and nurtures the gift of prophecy.

## IN CONCLUSION

The throat chakra is more complex than may at first appear. Its two distinct levels of functioning must always be taken into consideration.

Its Sanskrit name is 'Visuddha' and in classical Indian lore it is depicted as having sixteen petals, one for each of the Sanskrit vowels.

## MEDITATIONS AND SUGGESTIONS FOR WORKING WITH YOUR THROAT CHAKRA

### 1.  Contacting and Sensing Your Throat Chakra

Check the location of your throat chakra on the diagram on page 5. Then use the sensing exercise on page 36, substituting 'throat' where appropriate. Follow this with the 'Images and Symbols' exercise on page 37.

### 2.  Guided Visual Meditation for the Throat Chakra

Make sure that you are likely to be undisturbed . . . find a comfortable position for your body . . . let it be balanced, but relaxed . . . close your eyes and be in touch with the rhythm of your breathing . . . enter your own inner space . . . there is no landscape, but you are surrounded by colour . . . deep blues . . . aquamarines . . . and silver. . . . They give you a feeling of refreshment and lightness . . . at first you absorb them . . . then you begin to dance gently. . . . As you do so, the colours move . . . ripple . . . and dance with you. . . . You feel lifted and then realize that you are floating with a great sense of safety and freedom. . . . It is as though the colours hold you and surround you and your body is as light as the colours themselves . . . relax and give yourself up to the experience until you find that you can float and fly, free as a bird in the air currents, dipping and gliding . . . controlled . . . yet light. . . . You discover that you can choose a colour on which to float. . . . It may be one of the blues . . . aquamarines . . . or silvers. . . . It may be a different colour which has come into your inner world . . . let the world of colour and the particular colour of your choice, wrap itself around you ... go on a journey into colour ... maybe there is a boat in which to glide in this coloured world ... or a large fantastic bird or magic carpet on which to ride ... perhaps you just enjoy lightness, freedom and dance as you allow yourself to be carried along.... Eventually you come to a place of rest ... there are silky, cushioning clouds of the colour of your choice.... You relax into them and are still ... all movement has ceased ... there is a deep silence ... the most profound stillness you could ever have imagined, around you and within you.... You are centred, still and at one.... Soon, with a clarity which could only come after such a silence, you hear a single beautiful note ... pure, as though played on a magical flute, it comes from a distance ... softly at first ... building up to a pleasant intensity ... surrounding you ... so that you are aware of all its tones, undertones and overtones.... It is a healing sound ... it is around you ... it is in your body ... it is in your being.... As you relax into it, change comes once more ... you hear a whole orchestra of harmonious sounds, and you start to move again, on sound waves.... Let yourself be carried ... moving from one to another ... becoming part of a world of harmony.... You find that you are making a sound ... a rounded note, in your throat chakra ... you sing it or sound it ... it adds to the harmony around you and echoes back to you.... In this inner space you are capable of making a sound which you may not be able to make in the outer world ... you know that you will remember it and be able to attune to it as your special healing sound.... When you are ready to return, your special colour, bird, or boat will help you.... Travel back, until you come to the place where this journey began.... With your feet lightly in touch with the ground, the blue, aquamarine and silver colours surround you ... gradually you return to the awareness of the rhythm of your breathing ... to the awareness of your body and its contact with the ground in your everyday world.... Visualize a cross of white light, in a circle of white light over your throat chakra and draw a cloak of light with a hood right around you, as you return.

## 3.  Questions

Contemplate the questions 'How do I hear the world?' and 'How does the world hear me?'

## 4.  Fragrances

Use the fragrances for this chakra, to activate, calm, or balance it. See pages 33 – 5 for directions and suggestions for working with fragrances.

## 5.  Colours

Breathe into your throat chakra and 'feed' it with the colours given on page 87. Remember to visualize translucent colours, as stained glass appears when sunlight passes through it. Close down the petals of the chakra and visualize the cross or star of light in a circle of light over it to finish.

## 6.  Getting in Touch with the Developmental Age

Reflect on the period of your life between fifteen and twenty-one years old. Try to see how this period in particular may have affected your freedom to choose. What sort of things block your choices now – circumstances, money, family commitments, ability, training? Is there any way in which you could alter the *style* of some of the things which you dislike in your life but cannot change? For example: (a) An office worker who felt artistically frustrated in a mundane and sterile environment began to introduce colour, flowers, a cushion or so here and there and focused on making things more harmonious and fresh. People began to comment, depression lifted and, though the job did not change, each day was less stressful or dreaded; (b) When I felt stuck in teaching and longed to become a healer and counsellor, I managed to overcome the frustration of waiting by concentrating on all the ways in which teaching can be seen as healing.

## 7.   The Sense of Hearing

Make a special effort to listen to all the sounds around you.
Listen to the quality of your own, your partner's, children's,
or friends' voices. Make a tape recording of your own voice
and hear yourself as others hear you.

## 8.   Mantra, Chants and Affirmations

In the East mantra have been used for as long as religions
have existed. They are combinations of words which make
holy or sacred sounds and express a spiritual truth. The
Sanskrit mantram, 'Om Mani Padme Hum' (the jewel in the
heart of the lotus) is well known. The many names of God
may be chanted or sung ritualistically, or one of them may be
used, like the Sanskrit 'Om Namah Shivayah'. The
Japanese 'Namya Ho Ren Ge Kyo' expresses reverence for
creation and the Buddha nature. Often much of the effect lies
in the *sound* which builds up from repetitive singing or
chanting. Such practices heighten awareness, bring inner
stillness and aid focus and concentration, they induce
meditation and are expressions of worship and reverence.

A mantram in one's own language may have a slightly
different effect, because there is a more direct understanding
of the words, but repetition of a phrase one loves can enhance
meditation or contemplation. Some to try are:

Peace within
Abide with me
Be still and know
Father/Mother Creator
And the greatest of these is love
At one
Light from the Source
Be still my heart, one day we shall be one

The choice is wide, with many possibilities. The mantra may
be repeated mentally, spoken aloud, chanted or sung.

There is a revival of American Indian sung chants such as 'The river is flowing, flowing and growing, the river is flowing, down to the sea. Mother earth carry me, a child I shall always be, mother earth carry me, down to the sea.'

I have reservations about affirmations such as 'Every day, in every way I am getting better and better'. Though some people find them helpful, my concern is that they can come from, and work at, a mental level, masking the need to make a deeper emotional shift. If that shift has been made, then I believe that affirmations are a great help in retraining thought patterns and for building confidence.

## 9.   The Prayer or Affirmation

Meditate and reflect on the words given on page 87.

# Chapter 8

# The Brow Chakra

**Location**  Above and between the eyes, with a stem at the back of the head.

**Key Words**  Spirit, Completeness, Inspiration, Insight, Command

**Colours**  Indigo, Turquoise, Mauve

**Element**  Radium

**Body**  Higher Mental

**Glandular Connection**  Pineal

**Quietening Fragrances**  White Musk, Hyacinth

**Stimulating Fragrances**  Violet, Rose Geranium

**Crystals and Gemstones**  Amethyst, Purple Apatite, Azurite, Calcite, Pearl, Sapphire, Blue and White Fluorite

## Prayer or Affirmation

We seek to command ourselves through the inspiration of the command of God. May true insight be enabled and the finite mind be inspired to a knowledge of completion.

## Brow Chakra Case History

Eleanor is the busy mother of twin boys, who are now five years old. When she married, she was working as an occupational therapist and continued to do so until her pregnancy. She had always wanted children, so was not too shocked at the news that she was expecting twins. She prepared excitedly for their birth. Her husband, Michael, loved this time too. Among other things, he enjoyed her being at home for him when he returned from his commuter day.

Once the babies were born, Eleanor had little help and could not afford to employ anyone. She and Michael had an exhausting, though fulfilling, six months as they coped with the twins and all the life-changes which babies bring with them. Then Michael was offered a job with a big salary increase. This meant moving house, which was not easy with the twins just reaching the crawling stage, but they managed. In the new home, Eleanor could afford to have a cleaning lady. Michael did not have so far to travel to work and they could afford regular outings and baby sitters. They took great pleasure in creating their new home and in planning and planting the garden. They made local friends and were contented with life.

Settled in their new home, as the boys grew less demanding, Eleanor noted that sometimes she felt 'bored'. The usual round of playgroup events, barbecues with friends and even the evenings out with her husband took on a 'sameness' and lack of meaning. Her energy flagged. Her zest for living fluctuated. The doctor diagnosed mild depression and recommended a holiday without the children. Eleanor's mother was delighted at the opportunity to have her lively grandchildren to stay, and Eleanor and Michael went for a 'winter sun' holiday. This had been something they'd often dreamed about and which they visualized as being a second honeymoon. Eleanor enjoyed and benefited from the break but, once back at home, questions about the meaning of life began to nag at her. She became moody and irritable.

When the twins started full-time at school, Eleanor thought about going back to work for a couple of days a week. Michael did not see this as the answer. He was concerned about her health and wanted to protect her from stress. A friend suggested that she should try a complementary therapy, such as acupuncture. It was in the waiting room of the natural health clinic that Eleanor saw an advertisement for one of my workshops.

The whole spiritual concept was new to her. She had never been to a workshop before. At the first one she confessed to the group that she was 'terrified'. By the end of the day she could not wait for the next. New doors began to open for Eleanor. She made new friends with whom she could share experiences and discuss the new books she was reading. Learning about the chakras delighted her. She found that working with the brow chakra heightened her spiritual perceptions and provided access to her inner resources. She came to me for a few private sessions and learned to work with the colours, the stimulating oils and the other brow chakra exercises. (See pages 111 – 14.)

There were no dramatic changes of direction for Eleanor. She was one of those people whom the psychologist Jung described as 'discontent with being normal'. She had hidden spiritual resources, and by developing them found the greater meaning and purpose in life which had been lacking before.

People like Eleanor often feel guilty. In so many ways they know their lives to be blessed and fulfilled. They may have all kinds of material securities, but some key to happiness evades them. Sometimes they throw themselves into lives of service and sacrifice, neglecting partners, children and other commitments in order to do so. Opening the brow chakra can bring completeness, inspiration, insight and a sense of having command over one's own being.

# THE KEY WORDS

## Spirit

According to its nature, 'spirit' is difficult to define. It is often confused or contrasted with 'soul'. Gildas' teaching follows that of the spiritual alchemists where spirit is seen as yang and soul as yin (see *Gildas Communicates* in *Bibliography*). One of the aims of alchemy is to effect a mystical marriage between spirit and soul. Spirit is thus seen as clear, direct and initiating, while soul is receptive and gestating. The spirit initiates and commands life and its evolutionary tasks; the soul receives and sifts the experience gained. The spirit seeks completeness, commands action to enable it, and fertilizes inspiration and insight.

Within each one of us there is a spark or essence which never gets clouded. Somewhere, beyond our behaviour patterns and reactions to life, untouched by flaws of personality, character or morality, even within the most apparently vicious criminal, this spark burns on. When we know it in ourselves and honour it in others, it is near impossible to be inhumane.

Eleanor's unease was due to the spark of her spirit making itself known. Because of this her brow chakra had already started to open. She needed help in the conscious controlling, understanding and enjoyment of that opening.

## Completeness

As a key word for this chakra, it speaks of the urge to achieve perfection and wholeness. The brow centre awakens a need to enjoy the completeness of inner harmony of body, mind, emotions, spirit and soul.

## Inspiration

This may seem self-explanatory, in the sense of being spiritually inspired, or receiving inspiration. Yet this word also means 'in-breath'; the Greek 'pneuma' and the Latin 'spiritus' mean both spirit and breath. From such derivations came the Christian emphasis on the 'Breath of God', which we breathe in to inspire and animate us spiritually, physically and mentally.

## Insight

Insight links perception with understanding. It is the highest level of intuition. On the subtle levels, insight penetrates beyond the boundaries of time and space and enables a wider comprehension of the inner worlds and mysteries. When insight is activated in the brow centre, meeting with discarnate guides will be facilitated.

## Command

In Sanskrit, the name for the brow centre is 'Ajna', which literally translated, means 'command'. Through awakening this centre we can attain greater command of our lives and respond with enhanced awareness and sensitivity to the 'command' of our spirit.

# THE COLOURS

Indigo is a colour we find difficult to perceive and describe. It is fully present in any rainbow or spectrum, but more difficult to identify than the other more basic colours. Indigo dyes come from the indigo plant and are often used in West Indian batik work. The colour is neither purple, nor navy blue. It is intense and deep, sometimes almost black, but always containing a touch of red. Learning to differentiate indigo is, in itself, a good exercise for opening and awakening the brow chakra.

Mauve at the brow centre, is dark in tone. It is a hue between lavender and purple. Turquoise is the colour of the gemstone of the same name. It is bright and full bodied.

Use indigo to train perception, turquoise for clarity and mauve for helping the hormonal system.

## THE ELEMENT

Radium is a metallic, radio-active element used in X-rays, radio-therapy and the production of luminous materials.

Radio-therapy is well known for its use in the treatment of cancer and other tumours. It breaks down established patterns and brings about change. It is a radical treatment and all forms of radiation have well-known dangers. When Gildas was asked about radium he said: 'Radium brings power and light. It has a place in breaking down patterns in order to enable reassembly. It has a high vibrational rate. Its symbolism at the brow centre is about the facility of functioning on more than one level or dimension, while physically incarnate. It is about the meeting point of light and spirit in matter.'

## THE BODY

The higher mental body is of a supremely light and subtle substance. It reflects deep indigo and amethyst colours. It is the 'garment' which we wear for our highest levels of meditational experience, communication with other planes and at moments of inspiration.

The mental plane is one of pulsating energies. The inspiration which gives birth to ideas originates here, before it becomes clothed with language or form. It is the plane of divine principle, pure archetypal impulses and of the archangelic beings: Michael, Uriel, Raphael and Gabriel.

## THE GLANDULAR CONNECTION

Comparatively little is known about the pineal gland. It is located in the area found by taking a cross section immediately above the ears and centrally down from the top of the head. It is tiny, with a form resembling that of a pine cone. It is not yet known whether the pineal gland is part of the endocrine system or not. It secretes the hormone-like substance known as melatonin which, in animals, triggers the mechanisms of breeding and nesting cycles and the timing of migration and hibernation.

In humans, the pineal gland is light sensitive and controls our internal day and night 'clock'. There are nerve pathways between the pineal and the retina (in the eye). Current research is exploring the connection between the pineal gland, its supply of light and the control of body calcium levels.

Whether the pineal is part of the endocrine system or not, its relationship to light affects hormone levels. Blind people often suffer hormone imbalance, but if their sight is restored, normal hormone levels usually return. Working with the brow chakra can help with hormonal balance. Almost everything we do bears a hormonal stamp. Hormones regulate basic drives and emotions, sexual urge and identity, violence, anger, fear, joy and sorrow. They promote growth, control temperature, assist in the repair of broken tissue and help to generate energy.

## THE FRAGRANCES

White musk and hyacinth quieten this chakra, while violet and rose geranium stimulate it. Eleanor's brow chakra needed stimulation so that she could open to the spiritual side of life. Anxiety about spiritual progress and over-zealous use of meditation or other spiritual practices can lead to over-stimulation of the brow chakra. Growth of this kind cannot be forced and headaches above, behind and between the eyes may ensue. In such cases the quietening fragrances prove an effective treatment. They do not close a chakra down, but help its flow and movement to become calmer and steadier.

# THE CRYSTALS AND GEMSTONES

Information on how to work with crystals and gemstones can be found on pages 174 – 7.

☆ *Amethyst* used at the brow chakra promotes altered states of consciousness. It enhances spiritual awareness and encourages visionary qualities. It is a protective stone and transforms that which is negative.

☆ *Purple Apatite* stimulates all levels of perception. It encourages harmonious and peaceful inner work and aids meditation.

☆ *Azurite* is useful for rituals and blessing ceremonies as one of its qualities is sacredness. It promotes visionary dreams and awareness of the relationship between spirit and matter.

☆ *Calcite* helps to strengthen the higher mental body. It nurtures and promotes spiritual inspiration and experience. It links the world of spirit with the world of intellect and ideas.

☆ *Pearl* is a purifying stone. It creates an aura of serenity and aids devotion.

☆ *Sapphire* strengthens spiritual awareness and communication. It facilitates communication with guides and angels.

☆ *Blue Fluorite* is protective. It is a psychic shield, valuable in developing transcendent states of consciousness.

☆ *White Fluorite* strengthens the incarnate spirit. It helps to prevent depression and disillusionment.

## IN CONCLUSION

The brow is the penultimate chakra in every system – sevenfold, eightfold or twelvefold. It is the second in the subgroup formed by the throat/brow/crown. It does not have a dual function in the same way as the throat chakra but has an important connection with the solar plexus, since both are connected with light and vision. The brow helps to strengthen the relationship between the personality and the spirit.

In Indian systems it has two petals. At this level the simplicity in the number of petals shows a major increase in vibrational rate. The movement is so fast as to make that which is complex appear simple. Because the root chakra has the lowest vibrational rate its specific number of petals can most easily be seen. The faster the movement the more difficult it becomes to count petals, so two is used to represent a vast and uncountable amount. The Sanskrit name is 'Ajna' – meaning that it perceives and commands.

## MEDITATIONS AND SUGGESTIONS FOR WORKING WITH YOUR BROW CHAKRA

### 1. Contacting and Sensing Exercise for the Brow Chakra

Check the location of the brow chakra on the diagram on page 5. Then use the sensing exercise described earlier on page 36 substituting 'brow' where appropriate. Follow this with the 'Images and Symbols' exercise on page 37.

### 2. Guided Visual Meditation for the Brow Chakra

Make sure that you will be undisturbed. Sit or lie comfortably with your body balanced and symmetrically arranged. Pay particular attention to the comfort and balance of your head. Close your eyes and observe the rhythm of your breathing

. . . let this rhythm help you to focus your attention into your brow chakra . . . . Get an image of the petals of the chakra opening and relaxing . . . try to sense or visualize the pulsation and the circular movement of the chakric energy . . . enter your inner space and find yourself in a misty landscape, where it is either dawn or dusk. . . . Colours are undefined but objects are silhouetted against the horizon. . . . The air is fresh. . . . Despite the mistiness around, you feel innerly focused and clear. . . . Through the mist you can perceive hills . . . one, which is almost a mountain, attracts you . . . you find a gently winding path which takes you upwards . . . you become encompassed in a world of your own as the colours of indigo, turquoise and mauve swirl around you. . . . Within this undefined and surreal landscape you find it possible to be in touch with the deeper levels of your being. . . . You contact a sense of completeness and self-acceptance. . . . As the path winds on upwards any current problems which need resolving may take on a new perspective . . . you may feel creatively inspired. . . . The mist is clearing now and you realize that you are coming to a view-point over the landscape. . . . Mountain peaks rise into a clear turquoise sky . . . and beneath you the landscape gradually reveals itself. . . . You breathe in the clear air. . . . Suddenly, quite near to you, light is reflected from water with an unmistakable sparkle. . . . You go to explore and find a clear pool in a hidden and protected place . . . you look into it . . . where the light strikes the water in the centre of the pool there is an image of a flame . . . it seems to burn from the pool's depths and you are drawn more deeply into meditation. . . . Gradually you experience a quality which you know to be that of your in-dwelling spirit. . . . You may want to bathe in the pool . . . to immerse yourself in this quality and to relish the renewal which it can bring to every aspect of your being. . . . Whether you bathe or not, bask in this essence . . . allow insight to reveal new understanding of your life meaning and purpose. . . . When you are ready to return, trace the same path along which you came ... know that once you have found a place in your inner landscape you can always revisit it.... Draw the quality of your in-dwelling spirit around you like a mantle ... gradually become aware again of the rhythm of your breathing ... the contact of your body with the chair or ground ... take deep breaths ... put your feet firmly on to the ground ... open you eyes ... stretch ... arrive fully back into the outer world.... Visualize the petals of your brow chakra gently closing in ... put a cloak of light with a hood right around you.... Go about your normal daily tasks feeling refreshed and revitalized.

### 3. Fragrances

Use the particular fragrances for this chakra to activate it, calm it or balance it. See pages 33 – 5 for further directions and suggestions for working with fragrances.

### 4. Colours

'Breathe' into your brow chakra and 'feed' it with its colours, given on page 103. Remember to visualize the colours as translucent and to close down the petals and picture the cross or star of light in a circle of light over the chakra to finish.

### 5. Other Suggestions

(a) Find something beautiful to contemplate. If it is possible, go to an area of natural beauty. Take a beautiful object with you or read a poem, consider a picture or listen to some music. As you contemplate or listen, endeavour to be in touch with an essence of beauty. Try to acknowledge the spirit which can be released from matter and the spirit which can be expressed in matter.

(b) Contemplate the journey of your life, with all its positive and negative milestones. Try to recognize, without false pride or false modesty, the times where you acted from a spirit of inner integrity in times of opposition or difficulty.

(c) Search for something which is indigo coloured. Deep-coloured amethyst stones have touches of indigo in them. Try to train yourself to store this colour in your colour memory. Become more aware of the incidence of indigo in the environment, particularly in sunsets and other aspects of nature.

## 6.   The Prayer or Affirmation

Meditate and reflect on the words given on page 103.

# Chapter 9

# The Crown Chakra

**Location**   At the top of the head, with petals facing upwards and a stem going down into the central column.

**Key Words**   Soul, Surrender, Release, Incoming Will

**Colours**   Violet, White, Gold

**Element**   Magnetum

**Body**   Soul, Ketheric or Causal

**Glandular Connection**   Pituitary

**Quietening Fragrances**   Rosemary, Bergamot

**Stimulating Fragrances**   Violet, Amber

**Crystals and Gemstones**   Diamond, White Tourmaline, White Jade, Snowy Quartz, Celestite

## Prayer or Affirmation

Through surrender and release, let the incoming will be truly the will of God working within us and through us and leading us increasingly to knowledge of mystical union and mystical marriage.

## Crown Chakra Case History

Leo had recently retired after spending all his working life in social services. His career had been successful and satisfying. Quite early on, he had recognized a sense of vocation in helping people who were overwhelmed by life's problems or misfortunes. Tragedy in his own life had increased his empathy for others. He had married a fellow social worker and been blissfully happy for a brief eighteen months. Despair and devastation followed when his pregnant wife was killed in a car accident. Leo flung himself totally and intently into his work, suppressing almost all other interests. He did not remarry.

Despite, or perhaps because of, his misfortune, Leo had long been interested in spiritual matters. Some years before his retirement he realised that he would have to prepare carefully for it, since his work was his life. He saved money, and bought a house in the country, which he stocked with a comprehensive library. He made sure that he would have a comfortable pension and began to look forward to the time when he would live more quietly and make a deeper study of his books. At this point our paths crossed, when he came to receive guidance from Gildas.

Having carefully planned the end of his working life, Leo now wanted to discover a new sense of purpose for the active years still lying ahead. He was seeking spiritual fulfilment.

In his social work, Leo had been inspired by the throat chakra quality of vocation, magnified by his unfortunate loss. In finding a deeper meaning to life his brow chakra had become active. Now he needed to move more consciously into the crown energies, so as to fulfil and understand more of the total purpose and pattern of his life.

A fascination for Egyptology had survived even when Leo had shut so much out from his life. Gildas suggested that he should now concentrate on this interest and consider writing about ancient Egyptian social organization. He also gave Leo some meditations and exercises for the crown chakra, similar to those on pages 123 – 5.

Leo believed in reincarnation. As he proceeded with the deeper study which would precede his writing, he felt a sense of continuity. Perhaps he had been an Egyptian scribe or even a priest/healer? It was difficult for him to describe the sense of peace, release and surrender which entered his life from a relatively simple adjustment. He has found a new and satisfying path. Sometimes when he leaves his country retreat to come to London for his research, he visits me for a session or attends a workshop. He is invariably cheerful and enthusiastic and feels that the jigsaw pieces of his evolutionary and experiential spiritual journey are slotting gratifyingly together.

## THE KEY WORDS

### Soul

As defined by the spiritual alchemists, soul is yin, receptive and clouded by the burden of experience. Evolution progresses as the backcloth of the soul absorbs and reorganizes our actions and learning. The opportunity of reincarnation enables experience to be gained and balances to be made. The soul governs the pattern of karma and spurs into action its law of cause and effect. When the karmic journey nears its end the soul becomes a clear chalice in which the spark of the spirit can burn as a strong flame. This image represents the consummation of the mystical marriage and the birth of knowledge, light, vision, healing and wisdom.

### Surrender

This needs to be seen as graceful rather than abject. Leo, after the tragic loss of his wife, went through phases of grim surrender, over-compensation and angry rebellion before coming to a graceful acceptance of the pattern of his life. Retirement was more of a testing time for him than may immediately appear from the telling of his story. He needed the key which would bring the final special quality of surrender into his life, thus bringing spiritual contentment and completeness. Without reassurance or compensation he could have felt embittered, rebellious and rejected by life in his later years.

## Release

Release helps to prevent surrender from being a condition of blind obedience. It signifies a trust in the higher self which enables a relaxed attitude to life without a total abdication of responsibility and alertness.

## Incoming Will

This refers to the purposes of the soul for the present incarnation. When the lower will is able to release some of its intractability and surrender to the incoming will, then life becomes more harmonious and spiritually directed. These accomplishments are not possible except through the crown chakra. If natural alliance with the incoming will is difficult, then conscious work with the crown chakra will help.

# THE COLOURS

Violet has the highest vibrational rate in the sevenfold spectrum of colour. It is the violet of emperors and royalty, deep, rich and regal. White symbolizes both innocence and perfection. It is the unwritten page, the untried innocent, the virgin bride, but also the colour of the highest initiate reflecting the purity which comes from the return to innocence after experience. Gold symbolizes the power of the sun and sacredness. It is the colour of a most precious metal and also symbolizes purity. It is sometimes considered to be the colour of the masculine principle, but at the crown chakra should be understood as pertaining to balanced and perfected wisdom.

Violet is a cleansing colour – visualizing it at the crown chakra will help to cleanse impurities from the energy field. White and gold help to encourage contact with your higher self and guides.

## THE ELEMENT

Magnetum is not found in any standard list of elements. In the physical sense it has yet to be discovered, but Gildas is not the only guide to have identified it as an element for the crown chakra. Its symbolic quality is unification. It signifies the wholeness experienced when body, mind, emotions and spirit are in harmony. It enhances our awareness of humanity as a corporate body. It promotes the healing of our relationship to the earth and all its life forms and encourages a sense of proportion.

## THE BODY

This layer of the auric field holds the imprint of the learning intentions we have made for this lifetime. Contacting it, through the crown chakra, will help us to see a higher pattern, purpose and direction for our lives.

The names soul, ketheric or causal are alternative names for this body. Ketheric implies a higher level of the etheric body – described at the sacral chakra as the subtle 'double' of the physical body. The ketheric body is an evolutionary imprint or reflection from the soul. In incarnation this layer can affect us through the subtle memories from other lives which cause us to react to positive or negative stimuli in ways which are not directly explicable in terms of our present life experience. Unexpectedly intense or so-called irrational fears, 'freefloating' anxieties, *déjà-vu* experiences and exceptional giftedness are all examples of the interpenetration of the causal body.

## THE GLANDULAR CONNECTION

The pituitary gland regulates the endocrine system; it is the conductor of the endocrine orchestra. It is tiny – being only pea-sized – but powerful. It has two lobes and hangs by a short stalk from the undercarriage of the brain in a small hollow behind the nose and between the eyes. Each lobe is really a separate gland. The anterior lobe is the controller because all its hormones, except the growth hormone, mastermind the function of the other endocrine glands. The posterior lobe secretes the hormones which are responsible for the contraction of the uterus during pregnancy and for initiating lactation. It also secretes the substance which helps the kidneys to regulate body fluid and the levels of sodium and potassium.

The complex functions of the pituitary shows that it is largely responsible for the sort of bodies we have and the way in which they function. The subject of body biochemistry and behaviour versus the effect of environmental factors has been a long and continuing debate among researchers, of whom few would accept factors associated with the purposes of the soul. Yet the link between the crown chakra and the pituitary gland opens the physical channels through which the purposes of the higher self can be reflected in bodily and behavioural patterns laid down by the 'accident' of birth.

## THE FRAGRANCES

The quietening fragrances should be used if you feel over-anxious about your soul purpose and 'getting it right'. Such tensions about the spiritual path can sometimes lead to serious and disabling stress conditions.

Leo's crown chakra needed some gentle stimulation. The stimulating oils may also be used if you note any tendency in yourself to be stubborn or wilful, often finally to your own disadvantage.

## THE CRYSTALS AND GEMSTONES

Information on how to work with crystals and gemstones can be found on pages 174 – 7.

☆ *Diamonds* symbolize perfection and clarity. They draw us towards our highest spiritual potential and encourage the higher will to illumine the personality.

☆ *White Tourmaline* encourages integrity. It facilitates the deeper understanding of spiritual surrender and obedience. It is a spiritually purifying stone and so promotes inner honesty and insight.

☆ *White Jade* helps in awakening the inner divine spark. It strengthens communication with the higher self.

☆ *Snowy Quartz* heals resentment and loneliness. It strengthens the Soul body, while at the same time encouraging us to 'keep our feet on the earth'.

☆ *Celestite* aids meditation. It heals and fortifies the petals of the crown chakra and gives it vitality. It awakens our desire to celebrate the spiritual aspects of life.

## IN CONCLUSION

The chakras are energetic stepping stones. As we move upwards, culminating at the crown chakra, the vibrational rate increases. Through the crown chakra we experience the highest states of meditation, and help ourselves to feel spiritually alive. Yet to work only with the higher chakras without knowledge of the others can be like taking hold of a high tension wire. After meditations which focus on the higher chakras, it is particularly necessary to take care to refocus fully into the material world. Only then do we bring the relaxing and refining benefits of meditation with us in such a way as to enable us to live more effectively in the world as it is.

In considering the brow and crown chakras it may seem as though spirit, soul and the higher self impose a preconceived and harsh destiny on to the struggling personality. Seeing the causal levels as judgemental and controlling may kindle the fire of rebellion. Alternatively, feeling it impossible to contact our higher sense of purpose, we may sink into a morass of indecision and lack of direction. 'Why don't I just know what I'm meant to do, so that I can get on with it?' is a common and complaining question. We feel as though the little personality alone has to find the power to perform tasks which are unclear or too difficult.

Positive contact with the brow and crown chakras enables a resolution of these conflicts by unblocking the channels which enable the personality to receive light, strength and joy from the Divine source. When the power from soul and spirit flows in, then no task has to be undertaken in the strength of the little ego alone and surrender is not a depersonalizing experience.

The crown chakra is sometimes called 'the thousand petalled lotus'. The halos, seen in illustrations around the heads of Jesus and the Saints, signify the fully developed and open crown chakra.

The classical Sanskrit name for the crown chakra is 'Sahasrara', meaning 'thousandfold' and referring to the number of its petals.

## MEDITATIONS AND SUGGESTIONS FOR WORKING WITH YOUR CROWN CHAKRA

### 1.  Contacting and Sensing the Crown Chakra

Check the location of your crown chakra on the diagram on page 5. Then use the sensing exercise described earlier on page 36, substituting 'crown' as appropriate. Follow this with the 'Images and Symbols' exercise on page 37.

### 2.  Guided Visual Meditation for the Crown Chakra

Making sure that you will be undisturbed, sit or lie comfortably with your body in a symmetrical position, with your back well supported if necessary. Pay particular attention to the balance of your head and neck as this helps in aligning the chakras. Close your eyes and be aware of the rhythm of your breathing.... Let this rhythm help you to focus your attention into your crown chakra ... sense the many petals of this pulsating centre ... sense its bowl-like shape and the light and colour which it both produces and receives from above.... Gradually enter your inner space ... and find yourself in a meadow.... Take the opportunity to look around ... to see the objects and colours ... to smell the fragrances ... to hear the sounds ... touch the textures ... and taste the tastes.... Beyond the meadow you are aware of hills and mountains.... As you look towards them you see that the sun is shining on a hill or mountain top and lighting up a beautiful temple there.... You can see the pathway leading from the meadow to that high temple and are drawn to make the journey to it.... You may choose a companion, talisman or power animal to accompany you.... Travel until you reach the outer courtyards of the temple which you now see in the distance.... There may be some ritual which you need to go through in the courtyards before you enter the temple, such as changing your clothes ... taking off your shoes ... washing yourself ... or leaving behind things you may be carrying.... When you are ready the temple door will be standing open for you.... Enter and explore the temple ... note its sounds or its quality of silence ... its fragrances ... its colours, textures and tastes ... find a place in which to sit in meditative or receptive mood ... ask to be made more aware of your connection to your soul and higher self.... Affirm or renew any resolutions you wish to make about your spiritual life.... A temple-server may come to offer you wine or water from a special cup.... You may be given a blessing or a gift.... When all the ceremony is over, it is time to leave.... Knowing that this temple is here, you may revisit it whenever you wish to reconnect to your higher self.... Collect any belongings which you left outside the temple, though you can also leave any unwanted luggage behind.... Go through the outer courtyards once more and then return to the meadow, and thence to the awareness of the rhythm of your breathing ... to the contact of your body with your chair ... to your feet firmly on the ground ... to full awareness of your outer world.... Protect and bless your crown chakra with a cross of light in a circle of light ... and surround yourself with a cloak of white light with a hood.

## 3.  Fragrances

Use the particular fragrances for this chakra to activate it, calm it or balance it. See pages 33 – 5 for further directions and suggestions for working with fragrances.

## 4.  Colours

'Breathe' into your chakra and 'feed' it with its colours given on page 115. Remember to visualize the colours as translucent and to close down the petals, and picture in your mind the cross or star of light in a circle of light over your crown chakra to finish.

## 5.  Getting in Touch with Your Higher Self

Follow the temple meditation again but while there ask your higher self to comment on a specific question you want to ask. You may get a comment in thought, words, pictures or symbols.

## 6.  The River of Life

Visualize a river, flowing from its source to the sea.... Imagine it as the river of your life.... Find a landing stage, where there is a boat ... note what kind of boat it is, and whether there is someone to steer it for you, or whether you will manage it yourself.... Take the boat upstream towards the source, and as you travel, allow significant life memories to come into your awareness.... When you get near to the source you may have to leave the boat safely anchored or moored and continue on foot.... At the source drink some water, and then sit and rest for a while.... As you rest you may be aware of companions ... those with whom you have a special connection and who were with you in essence as you started your life journey ... some of them will be in incarnation with you now ... others may not.... Try to get insight about your true companions on the evolutionary journey ... your spiritual family, who may not be the same as your genetic family.... When you are ready, return to your boat and down the river to your landing stage, leaving the boat safely tied and anchored there. Take time to draw or write about this journey and to consider any memories which were awakened. Is there some implicit message or pattern to bring you insight about the present phase of your life?

## 7.  The Prayer or Affirmation

Reflect or meditate on the words given on page 115.

# Chapter 10

# The Implications of the New Chakras

No matter how many chakras are seen as forming the major system, the crown remains the 'highest'. For a sevenfold scheme the exploration of the chakras is now complete. Yet Gildas and other channelled sources have suggested that there should be an expansion into twelve major centres rather than seven.

Many generations have anticipated a crisis or world change during their era. Apocalyptic beliefs generate fear and dread, yet often feed on guilt or inadequacy in the face of complex difficulties. Today we are better able to measure and quantify and so know how culpable we are of misusing resources and polluting the earth. Sophisticated communication systems make us more immediately aware of world problems and of 'man's inhumanity to man'. We realize that unless we can orchestrate some form of transformation, negative degeneration will take over. More people than at any other time in our history are demanding, instigating and responding to appeals for change. The old order is inadequate for the management of the foreseeable future in a way which it has never been before. The pace of technological discovery and its effects on material life is in a constant state of acceleration. Innovations are in danger of redundancy before they reach the end of the assembly line.

At the same time as the demand for change there is widespread depression, despair and hopelessness about the dimensions of the shift which is required. Individuals become discouraged when it seems that anything they can offer is but a drop in the ocean.

In Chinese the written word for crisis consists of two glyphs which, separated, mean 'danger' and 'opportunity'. We must not be complacent. Danger is certainly present, yet we also have an unprecedented opportunity to make the 'quantum leaps' in awareness which will enable us to move into a new and exciting phase of evolution.

In their teaching about 'new' chakras – the alter major, the base, the hara, the unconditional love centre and the third eye – the guides are showing us that we have the necessary resources of spiritual strength to make these quantum leaps. The expanded chakra system helps us to see how every drop in the ocean, no matter how small, is of great significance to the whole.

## Chapter 11

# The Alter Major Chakra

**Location** Petals in the area of the nose. Positive energy centre in its stem, which is where the back of the head begins to bend round, corresponding with the 'old' or 'lizard' brain, before the division into right and left hemispheres.

**Key Words** Instinct, Resonance, Duality, Devic Nature, Healing

**Colours** Brown, Yellow Ochre, Olive Green

**Element** Wet Earth

**Sense** Smell

**Body** Instinctual and Lower Causal

**Glandular Connection** Adrenals

**Quietening Fragrances** Musk, Cedarwood

**Stimulating Fragrances** Violet, Rose Geranium

**Crystals and Gemstones** Carnelian, Tiger's Eye, Snow Flake Obsidian, Fossils, Peacock Stone

### Prayer or Affirmation

Through engagement with our Devic Nature may we move from duality and split to oneness and unity.

## Alter Major Chakra Case History

I met James, a business executive, when I was working as counsellor and healer in a residential natural health centre. He had become severely stressed, and his blood pressure was dangerously high. He attended my daily relaxation classes and asked for some individual counselling sessions. His wife, Mary, was at the health centre too, giving James support and taking a much needed break herself. She was desperately concerned, and found her workaholic husband stressful to live with.

James found it difficult to relax. He was already wondering how to survive the remaining three weeks of the month for which he had booked. His 'normal' life consisted of a long commuter day. He took his lap-top computer and portable telephone everywhere with him. Every journey was spent working. When he went abroad, he never took Mary with him, or allowed extra time to see anything of the interesting places which he visited. In the evenings or at weekends he was always to be found at his desk.

James had a lovely house on the edge of the countryside, but never went for walks. He employed someone to help his wife with their large garden, rather than get involved himself. He was reluctant to take holidays and, when persuaded to do so, the lap-top and sheafs of papers invariably went with him. On the few occasions that his wife could persuade him to go to the theatre or to socialize with friends, he was restless, irritable and abrupt.

Mary said that James only went outside on his way to the car, train or plane. She was sure that he was unaware of the seasons of the year – he wore lighter shirts and suits in summer only because she put them out for him.

When I told James that I was a healer as well as a counsellor he was surprisingly open to 'trying it out'. Perhaps he thought I could weave some magic which would allow him to go back to his old ways without making himself ill. I decided to work principally on his alter major chakra, encouraging it to open. His energy field at the back of his head felt tight, static and numb. I did some guided imagery with him, emphasizing natural scenes and the elements. Foreseeably, James found visualization difficult but playing quiet background music helped and he actually began to enjoy our sessions.

James was not the sort of person who would work directly with his chakras, but I taught him to massage the alter major positive polarity point, gently, with his fingertips. The health centre had extensive grounds, with cows and horses in adjoining fields and access to the sort of woods where the leaf-mould is thick, and the scent of damp earth pervades. Mary encouraged James to walk in the woods with her and noticed that he was gradually becoming less restless and more able to converse with her in a relaxed way as they strolled through the greenery.

One day, Mary found James sitting on a bench, watching the cows chewing the cud. She sat near him and after a while he took her hand and said, 'All I really need to do is remember to watch cows more often.' It was a true turning point. The combined treatments at the health centre were effective. James left with a much lower blood pressure reading, a determination to change his life-style and a love of cows. Mary left with hope for the future quality of life and their marriage.

## THE KEY WORDS

### Instinct

Instinct was mentioned in connection with the root chakra. Working with the alter major can be instrumental in reawakening instinctual alertness. The energetic linking of this chakra to the old brain cortex, or 'lizard brain' puts us in touch with the non-verbal message system which protects

us from danger. This is similar to that which causes rats to
leave a ship or pit ponies to refuse to enter a coal-seam, well
in advance of any other warnings that something is wrong.
As humans, if we 'happen' to get up and leave the room just
before the ceiling falls in over the chair where we were sitting
we explain it away as 'lucky chance'. We say, 'my number
wasn't up yet', or 'my guardian angel was working hard'. It
is difficult for us to believe that these happenings come from
a non-verbal signalling which can be more consciously
cultivated. If this sense had not been so universally lost or
dishonoured, our planet might not now be facing imminent
disaster. Warnings tend only to be accepted if they have been
scientifically or intellectually 'proven'. Prophets working
intuitively or instinctually are not respected and may even
become figures of fun.

## Resonance

This is the phenomenon which Rupert Sheldrake (see
*Bibliography*) named 'morphic resonance'. Psychologists and
scientists are finding considerable evidence in favour of the
'hundredth monkey' theory being applicable to humans as
well as to animals. Thus one monkey on an island learns to
wash potatoes before eating them and then teaches another,
who teaches another. As soon as one hundred monkeys wash
potatoes, all monkeys everywhere will wash them without
having gone through the conscious learning process. (The
figure 'one hundred' represents an optimum number or
proportion.)

Jung wrote extensively about the 'collective unconscious'
(see *Bibliography*), theorising that everything which humans
do or have ever done affects and impinges on each one of us.
These energies suggest exciting possibilities for the role of the
individual in collective change. With sophisticated communication systems the 'optimum number' may be more
easily reached. In recent years world days of prayer, peace,
meditation and humour have played a considerable role
in changing our awareness and encouraging us to share

resources. What is not so universally known is that working with the alter major chakra increases the efficiency of morphic resonance and the 'creative minority'. When enough people know this, then quantum leaps will surely happen in our time.

## Duality and Devic Nature

These two key words have to be considered together. The alter major is the centre which strengthens our contact with plants, trees, animals, rocks, elements, seasons, growth cycles and the substance of earth itself.

When natural rhythms and cycles are observed, the whole of life becomes more harmonious, disease decreases and is healed more easily from natural resources. When, through lack of awareness, we interfere with the natural worlds, we foster duality and increase our vulnerability to deep levels of sickness which are resistant to healing.

Pan, the mythological king of the elemental worlds is the symbolic or *archetypal* figure for this chakra. His portrayal is a dual one, either as a young man playing the Pan pipes and calling forth abundance and fertility, or as half-goat, half-man, with an enormous erect phallus occasioning fear of rape and nightmare. In this guise he causes pan-ic or pan-demonium.

Comparatively little is known about the beings who are the energetic guardians of the elemental and natural worlds – they are variously called angels, devic beings, nature spirits, fairies, gnomes, elves, undines, nereids and sprites. They have long been portrayed in stories and illustrations as part of our mythical consciousness. Devas are guardians of rivers, valleys, hillsides and trees. Fairies, elves, undines and nereids are energy beings with a sense of fun. They appear to those who have 'the sight' in semi-human form when they want to attract attention and communicate. They are bewildered when we do not see their flashes of light and colour or hear the tinkle of their laughter. Where there is energy, there they are. When all is well they work with the devas and direct their energies towards growth, fertility and abundance. When things are out of balance they are drawn to wherever the energy flow is strongest. Formed of basic energy they are primitively amoral and will pick up on and accentuate difficult as well as positive animation or inter-action.

## Healing

Healing has an important association with devic nature. Within each one of us there is a natural or self-healing mechanism. Problems brought about by the dualities and oppositions of life often underlie the process of disease. Research shows that we can influence consciously the so-called autonomous systems of the body when we learn to activate the right side of the brain.

Although connected to the old brain cortex, the alter major is more in tune with the right brain than the left. (See *Glossary*.) When we engage deliberately with our self-healing mechanisms, the elementals within us are enabled to help our bodies back to health and harmony. A large factor in health or disease patterns is the balance of earth, air, fire and water within our bodily systems.

A positive relationship to all the alter major key words results in a deeper understanding of our health patterns. Instinct is an early warning system. Resonance and devic nature help us to take our rightful and harmonious place within the total pattern of the universe. Duality teaches us to make responsible choices.

## THE COLOURS

Even the denser colours of this chakra should be visualized as they would appear in a stained glass window with sunlight passing through. Each of the alter major colours is frequently found in nature and natural dyes. Ancient civilizations used them in their paintings and craftwork.

Brown is quite deep in tone with a touch of red. Yellow ochre is the colour of old mustard, often seen in lichens and tree fungi. Olive green in this chakra is the silvery green of the leaves of olive trees found in Provence and other Mediterranean areas. It is this colour, rather than the brighter shade of green olives, which should be used when visualizing for this chakra.

Visualizing the alter major colours will help to awaken this useful centre and to strengthen your relationship to the natural worlds. Yellow ochre aids the development of the instinctual, pre-verbal early-warning system.

## THE ELEMENT

Wet earth connects the alter major to the root and sacral chakras. Walking in woods which smelled of damp leaf-mould helped James to reconnect with nature and its fertile rhythms. Wet earth brings abundance from the natural cycles of death, decomposition and composting.

Wet earth is well-known by archaeologists for its preservative value.

Symbolically, this element represents the flow of knowledge in a continuous cycle from unconscious to conscious and back again. Everything humanity has learned or experienced cannot be held in uppermost awareness all the time, it has a cadence as natural as that of the seasons of the year or the sap of trees. In sinking back into its storage places it is fertilized and reactivated and when it rises again brings rebirth and new growth.

## THE SENSE

This is the same as for the root chakra and is described on page 30.

# THE BODY

The lower causal is a layer within the soul, ketheric or causal body. (See page 119.) It is that part of the subtle energy field which governs the rhythms chosen by the soul. Our birth will happen at a specific time, and we will be preserved from death until our agreed life span has been reached. Awareness of, and communication with, this level of our beings, brings about a more immediate working out of the karmic laws of cause and effect, leaving less unfinished business to be balanced out in a future lifetime.

# THE GLANDULAR CONNECTION

This is the same as for the solar plexus. (See page 68.)

# THE FRAGRANCES

Some people are so attuned to the elements and natural earth rhythms that they seem almost like sprites in appearance and movement or in a 'butterfly' attitude to life. In these cases the alter major chakra may be disproportionately active and the quietening fragrances are needed.

James's alter major chakra was quite tightly closed. His masseur at the health clinic added a mixture of lavender and amber oils to the usual massage oil.

# THE CRYSTALS AND GEMSTONES

Information on how to work with crystals and gemstones can be found on pages 174 – 7.

☆ *Carnelian* encourages contact with nature spirits. It aids memory of previous life times and the dreaming of 'great dreams'.

☆ *Tiger's Eye* enables greater contact with the earth and its rhythms and seasons. It will aid the growth of planted herbs when shallowly buried among them.

☆ *Snow Flake Obsidian* is linked to the cycles of death and rebirth and brings us stamina for all times of change. It strengthens the instinctual/lower causal body.

☆ *Fossils* help us to connect to the wisdom stored in the collective unconscious. They promote a natural and relaxed approach to life, incarnation and evolution.

☆ *Peacock Stone* (sometimes called Bornite or Chalcopyrites) aids the recall of skills which have been known and practised in another lifetime, or which are stored in the collective unconscious. This particularly applies to the revival of ancient healing skills.

# IN CONCLUSION

An 'alta' major chakra is described in the writings of Alice Bailey. (See *Bibliography*.) 'Alta' means 'higher', whereas 'alter' means 'other'. Some Eastern yogic systems also include a chakra at the back of the head which is not related to a specific number of petals or to the Sanskrit vowel sounds, as are the seven classical chakras.

With the other seven chakras there is a sequential progression from lower to higher, according to their vibrational rate and their position in relationship to the upright human body. The placement of the alter major is thus out of sequence. Although situated between the throat and the brow, its vibrational rate comes between those of the root and sacral chakras. Its element is a combination of earth and water; it shares the sense of smell with the root chakra and its glandular connection is the same as for the solar plexus.

# MEDITATIONS AND SUGGESTIONS FOR WORKING WITH YOUR ALTER MAJOR CHAKRA

## 1.  Contacting and Sensing the Alter Major Chakra

Remember that the alter major has its positive polarity (in the magnetic sense), in its stem. Its energy thus flows from back to front.

Use the sensing exercise described on page 36 substituting 'alter major' where appropriate and follow with the 'Images and Symbols' exercise on page 37.

## 2.  Guided Visual Meditation for the Alter Major Chakra

Making sure that you will be undisturbed, sit or lie comfortably. Close your eyes and aided by the rhythm of your breathing enter that state of relaxation where you can visualize your inner landscape and find yourself walking through a wood. . . . It is cool, shady and damp and there is a thick carpet of soft, loamy leaf-mould underfoot. . . . You have entered the wood from the hot sunshine beyond, and the shady coolness feels good . . . the scents of trees, plants and hidden animals are very strong. . . . The pathway is winding, but is obviously leading you to the centre of the wood. . . . Here and there you see ancient rocks, covered with moss and lichen. . . . You see a complete 'fairy ring' of toadstools and realize that this is a very special and magical place. . . . The trees are gradually becoming less dense . . . more light is filtering through, and soon you come into a clearing. . . . As you enter it, you are dazzled for a moment by the brightness of the sun after the shade of the wood. . . . As you focus again, you see an ancient stone circle here. . . . Around the stones the grass is green and lush . . . there is a special quality of silence. . . . You walk around the circle, touching each of the stones with a sense of awe and reverence for their age . . . after a while you find a place to sit, with your back resting against one of them ... your stone has been warmed by the sun.... There is a sense of timelessness as warm, healing energy pours into your spine.... You feel the deep connection of these stones with the earth which has supported their long standing.... You become aware of their resonance with each other, as they form their sacred circle.... You wonder about the ancient people who had the wisdom and earth knowledge to place these stones here.... Soon, strengthened, healed and warmed, you take one last walk around the circle, touching each stone again and feeling its texture ... then you take your leave ... walk back through the cool damp wood ... into the sunshine beyond it ... back to an awareness of the rhythm of your breathing and of your body.... Put your feet firmly on the ground and come back fully into your everyday world.... Surround yourself with a cloak of light with a hood, and visualize a cross or star of light in a circle of light over the back and front of your alter major chakra.

### 3.   Fragrances

Use the particular fragrances for this chakra, to activate it, calm it or balance it. See pages 33 – 5 for further directions and suggestions for working with fragrances.

### 4.   Colours

'Breathe' into your alter major chakra (from back to front) and 'feed' it with its colours given on page 128. Remember to picture in your mind the cross or star of light in a circle of light over both the front and the back of this chakra to finish.

### 5.   Other Suggestions

(a) Find out about some of the ancient festivals for honouring the rhythms of the earth, and her seasons (see *Bibliography*). Gather friends and/or family and do something to celebrate one of these days.
(b) Become more aware of the four elements – earth, water, fire and air – by taking walks in natural places and

by observing the part they play in our lives and in our bodies.

(c) Become more aware of the animal kingdom. Renew your appreciation of any pets or animals with whom you have contact. Listen to the taped sounds of dolphins or whales.

(d) Appreciate your sense of smell more. Using the fragrances will help here, but become more aware of the pleasant and unpleasant smells around. Make a special effort to use natural fragrances, such as lavender or pot pourri, in your home or work environment.

(e) Renew your appreciation of your garden or house plants. See if anything needs composting or repotting.

(f) Using your fingertips, and a gentle stroking movement, massage the positive polarity point of your alter major chakra at the back of your head.

## 6. The Prayer or Affirmation

Reflect or meditate on the words given on page 128.

# Chapter 12

# The Base Chakra

**Location**   Petals over the pubic bone, stem at the coccyx

**Key Words**   Retribution, Redemption, Choice, Transition, Peace, The World

**Developmental Age**   Conception to Birth

**Colours**   Deep Rose Red, Ruby, Purple

**Element**   Earth

**Body**   Causal

**Quietening Fragrances**   Heather, Rosewood

**Stimulating Fragrances**   Lemon Verbena, Thyme

**Crystals and Gemstones**   Rhodocrosite, Moonstone, Rose Quartz, Rose Opal, Rubilite

## Prayer or Affirmation

We acknowledge the interaction of our soul choice for retribution with our psychological environment. We seek to understand and surrender to the transition from retribution to redemption.

## Chakras with a Difference

This chakra, and the other three remaining, are newly awakening and, as such, cannot be given case-histories.

The base is the only new chakra with a developmental age. It is more directly related to the physical body than the hara, unconditional love centre, or third eye, but does not have a glandular connection.

Where people are only familiar with the sevenfold system, the root chakra may also be called 'the base'.

## The Key Words

### Retribution, Redemption and Choice

These refer to particular phases or types of karma. Before coming into incarnation we make choices, helped by our higher selves, guardian angels and guides. Gildas stresses the importance of 'retributive', 'redemptive' and 'transcendent' karma.

Before becoming incarnated, we decide, in consultation with our higher selves, the karmic lessons which need to be learned. We then choose the setting for life, and the factors which will affect our awareness and opportunities. If, for instance, we have misused power in another lifetime and made others our victims, we may incarnate into circumstances which are psychologically or physically disempowering. In struggling to overcome such a stumbling block we must learn to use power effectively. We might thus turn the setback to advantage by developing integrity and using it in our dealings with others.

When such change happens, we enter the redemptive phase of karma, where we consciously endeavour to turn our talents and learning to good use for humanity.

The transcendent stage of karma is when non-attachment has been learned, and there is graceful surrender to the higher will. (See page 122.)

These karmic phases do not have a linear or hierarchical progression. At any given time, in different areas of our lives, we may be dealing with all three.

## Transition

This applies to the period from just before conception, to birth. During this time the spirit is making the final preparations for incarnation. The higher self, guardian angel and guides oversee the journey.

## Peace and the World

Each of the new chakras has two archetypes as key words. The awakening base chakra will make us more eager to have peace in our world. It will move us more strongly to make the experience of being human one of solidarity and brotherly/sisterly love.

# THE DEVELOPMENTAL AGE

Recent years have seen much philosophical, spiritual and medical debate about the moment at which the human foetus can be said to be 'viable'.

Most discarnate guides agree that the spirit does not enter the foetus until just before or just after birth. During the gestation period, it draws very near, and the experiences of the foetus in the womb affect it greatly, but true incarnation, in the esoteric sense, only happens with birth.

During gestation, the soul and spirit become fully aware of the consequences of the choices which have been undertaken. Preparations for coming into the world as a helpless child are completed. From the higher perspective birth can seem like death, and death as rebirth.

# THE COLOURS

Deep rose red is the actual colour seen in the rose garden. It has great depth, with a quality of vulnerability or wounding within it. Ruby is the colour of the well-known gemstones, and of deep red wines. Purple is a slightly less brilliant hue than the violet of the crown chakra. It is denser in quality.

Ruby and purple are good colours for expectant parents to visualize around the mother's womb, to welcome the incoming being and give it a calm transition and incubation.

Deep rose red encourages an awareness of the earth, its vulnerability, its gifts and the need for a more positive relationship with it and its resources and its gifts.

# THE ELEMENT

This is the same as for the root chakra. When the base chakra is more fully awakened we shall become worthy to 'inherit the earth'. The message of this chakra is similar to those of the root and alter major. The key to its 'difference' or unique contribution lies in the word 'choice'. With greater awareness of the options we must take, we shall eventually retain more awareness of the spiritual worlds as we make the transition into incarnation. More children being born now have that distinctive 'old soul' look. This is related to a more active base chakra.

# THE FRAGRANCES

As this chakra is rarely developed enough to need quietening, for the present it is best to mix the four essences given on page 140 into a balancing fragrance as and when needed.

## The Crystals and Gemstones

Information on how to work with crystals and gemstones can be found on pages 174 – 7.

☆ *Rhodocrosite* has a gentle energy. It promotes our ability to love the earth and to recognize the interaction of spirit with matter.

☆ *Moonstones* chosen for use with the base chakra should be those which are very slightly pink in tone. They help us to make transitions and to move from retributive to redemptive karma.

☆ *Rose Quartz* is comforting. At this chakra it aids us to keep alive the connection with our guardian angel.

☆ *Rose Opal* facilitates birth. It is useful for mothers during labour, but also aids the birth of ideas and new phases of life or rites of passage.

☆ *Rubilite* assists our memory of the spiritual worlds and planes. It encourages us to incorporate beauty and sacred dimensions into the things we create and the buildings we build.

## Meditations and Suggestions for Working with Your Base Chakra

### 1.   Contacting and Sensing the Base Chakra

Use the exercise first described on page 36 substituting 'base' where appropriate. Follow this with the 'Images and Symbols' exercise on page 37.

### 2.   Guided Visual Meditation for the Base Chakra

Making sure that you will be undisturbed, sit or lie comfortably. Close your eyes and aided by the rhythm of your breathing enter that state of relaxation where you can visualize your inner landscape.... Find yourself sitting on a hilltop at night.... Warmth surrounds you and the air is pleasant ... the night sky is like diamond-studded velvet ... all the stars and the 'Milky Way' are clear ... the moon is bright, but still quite new .... Beneath you sparkle the lights of scattered houses or farms, for you are in a rural area.... Contemplate this view of the world, becoming aware of the towns and cities beyond ... the seas and rivers ... other continents and countries ... the roundness of the planet earth.... Project your awareness into space and imagine the view of our planet as seen by astronauts.... Be aware of the teeming life-force of humanity.... Reflect on the problem of suffering, but concentrate on a vision of a better world ... the potential family of humanity, giving and receiving love from each other, irrespective of colour or creed ... Return to your contemplation of the starry night sky.... In the distance, a shooting star zooms towards earth.... Reflect that some peoples believe a shooting star to be a soul on its way to, or from the earth ... a symbol of birth or death ... think of all who will be born or who will die this day ... bless their transition.... Gradually become aware of your breathing again ... be aware of your body.... Put your feet firmly on the ground ... and return fully to your everyday environment.... Let the petals of your base chakra close in, and put a cross or star of light in a circle of light over it as a blessing.

## 3. Fragrances

Blend the fragrances for this chakra to form a balancing mix. See pages 33 – 5 for further directions and suggestions for working with fragrances.

## 4. Colours

'Breathe' into your base chakra, and 'feed' it with its colours given on page 140. Remember to visualize the colours as translucent. Picture in your mind the cross or star of light in a circle of light over the chakra petals to finish.

## 5.   Other Suggestions

(a) Reflect on your life and see whether you can identify any of the stages of karma. What obstacles have you overcome, developing unexpected strengths in the process?

(b) Find out what influence may have affected you in the womb. Were you eagerly awaited – or was your imminent arrival beset by problems, changes, doubts or fears? Heal any wounding from this time, by imagining the journey of a totally welcome and excitedly awaited child.

(c) Contemplate the things in life which bring you peace. Resolve to make more space for these – soon.

## 6.   The Prayer or Affirmation

Reflect or meditate on the words given on page 140.

# Chapter 13

# The Hara Chakra

**Location** In the auric field between the sacral and solar plexus chakras.

**Key Words** Vitality, Power, Healing, Regeneration, Balance, God

**Colours** Apricot, Silver, Platinum

**Element** Granite

**Quietening Fragrances** Hibiscus, Apricot

**Stimulating Fragrances** Frankincense, Lily of the Valley

**Crystals and Gemstones** Honey Calcite, Sun Stone, Iron Pyrites 'suns', Stibnite, Wulfenite

## Prayer or Affirmation

We acknowledge and connect with the universal vital life-force. We accept our potential for health and regeneration, knowing that release from disease will bring collective self-actualization.

## INTRODUCING THE HARA CHAKRA

The chakras already explored have interpenetrated with the physical body. The hara does not. It has a vortex-like form and is situated away from the body, but contained within the aura. It has lines of energy connecting it to other major and minor chakras. The hara centre is naturally awake in some people, but quite closed, or barely discernible in others. The first step in gaining access to its vital and beneficial qualities is to work to strengthen its energetic connections. These links are to the sacral and solar plexus chakras, and to minor chakras over the liver and the spleen. When the connecting lines are developed they support the hara vortex and enable it to open and spin. Vitality reserves are then replenished naturally from the 'universal source' giving us stamina, high energy levels and the ability to 'bounce back' quickly following exertion or stress.

In Chinese models of the energy system there is a point or centre called the 'Chi'. Its location is similar to that of the hara.

## THE KEY WORDS

### Vitality

Vitality is the force which gives us zest for life and the ability to face each moment as it comes. It should not be confused with hyper-activity which is an unnatural state, and exhausts our adrenalin reserves. When we are near someone who is vital, we also feel refreshed, whereas those who are hyper-active exhaust themselves and those around them.

### Power

According to Chambers Dictionary, power is the 'ability to do anything – spiritual, mental, physical' and 'the capacity for producing an effect'. We often avoid the subject of power, tending to see it negatively. Certainly the experience of two world wars must make us aware of the truth of the saying 'absolute power corrupts'. Yet if we deny personal power we remain impotent in the face of opposition. We need to cultivate trust in our 'capacity for producing an effect' if we are not to sink into lethargy in the face of the difficulties of our era.

Power is an archetype of 'higher quality' and, as such, needs to be viewed positively.

## Healing

Many gifted healers work naturally from the hara centre. Using its strength helps them to avoid depletion and 'taking on' traces of patients' symptoms.

Self-healing capacity is also enhanced by developing the hara chakra and by linking with it when doing healing visualizations.

## Regeneration

Regeneration has been discussed on pages 51–2 in its relationship to the sacral chakra. The hara produces regenerative vitality.

## Balance

Balance given to us by this chakra is physical as well as symbolic. When the hara is active our physical balance and poise improve. Dancers usually have naturally developed hara chakras.

## God

God is the *second* archetype for this chakra. It can be argued that God is not strictly an archetype, since all archetypal energy emanates from the Source. Yet, religion has been a part of every known culture – even as early as Palaeolithic man. The drive to find spirituality in life and the common belief in a 'Creator' God or Divine Intelligence are generated by an archetypal impulse.

## THE COLOURS

Apricot is the colour of ripe apricots, soft and warm in tone. It enhances the body's ability to heal itself. Silver is the colour of the precious metal. In healing, it is used when flexibility with strength is required. Platinum is similar to silver, but rather more blue in tone. Symbolically it means stamina and endurance.

## THE ELEMENT

Granite is a very hard stone with quartz and silica in its constitution. It symbolizes the strength and stamina which the hara chakra gives.

## THE FRAGRANCES

Hyper-active people or children need the quietening fragrances to encourage the gentle flow of the hara energy. This chakra does not breed tension or hyper-activity but the stimulating fragrances encourage movement while the quietening ones bring composure.

People with fast-growing cancers can also benefit from use of the quietening fragrances.

Apart from the above exceptions, most of us need the help of the stimulating fragrances here. All four can also be mixed to make a balancing essence.

## THE CRYSTALS

Information on how to work with crystals and gemstones can be found on pages 174 – 7.

☆ *Honey Calcite* encourages balance. It helps in strengthening the energy supports which the hara needs for optimal functioning.

☆ *Sun Stone* facilitates receptivity to energy from the universal source. It stimulates self-healing abilities.

☆ *Iron Pyrites 'suns'* are comparatively rare forms of the pyrites family and are flat gold disks with shining rays coming from a central point. They facilitate resistance to stress.

☆ *Stibnite* is a useful crystal for healers. It has a metallic, striated appearance. It enables a steady flow of energy to others and helps in cultivating a calm, refreshing presence.

☆ *Wulfenite* is associated with the hara because of its apricot colouring. It strengthens the auric field. It helps all who are in positions of authority to temper power with compassion.

## MEDITATIONS AND SUGGESTIONS FOR WORKING WITH YOUR HARA CHAKRA

You will not find the hara chakra exercises easy until you have had considerable practice with those given for the other chakras.

### 1. Building the Energetic Structure

For this exercise, it is important to be sitting in an upright position, with your back supported if necessary. Use a cross-legged or lotus posture if you wish, but if sitting normally on an upright chair do not cross your legs or ankles.

Close your eyes and do the central column exercise for a few minutes (pages 7 – 8). Focus your attention into your sacral chakra and concentrate on letting its petals open flexibly. Move your awareness up, through the central column, to your solar plexus centre. Let these petals open also. Move your attention slightly upwards and to the right and locate the energy centre over your spleen, then get a sense of moving inwards, in relationship to your body, and find your liver centre.

Imagine spiralling strands of golden energy streaming from each of these centres into your auric field and meeting at a point in front of and above the sacral centre but below the solar plexus. Concentrate until you can feel this structure getting quite clear and strong. Working for a few minutes each day over a period of time will be more successful than trying too hard at a single session.

When the structure is well established you will naturally become aware of the hara vortex itself, opening, spinning and returning vitality through the spiralling lines of connection to the vital organs of the body. You do not need to close the hara chakra down, it will regulate itself according to your needs.

## 2.　Guided Visual Meditation for the Hara Chakra

Making sure that you will be undisturbed, sit or lie comfortably, close your eyes and, aided by the rhythm of your breathing, enter that quiet state in which you can withdraw into your inner space. Breathe your attention into that area of your auric field where your hara chakra is located ... see the chakra as a vortex of mingled apricot, silver and platinum colour ... become aware of the spiral patterns of energy in and around the hara vortex.... Feel as though you are entering a deep pool of strong but gently spiralling light.... Strength flows into you.... You feel safely warmed by the apricot light ... the silver brings a sense of clarity ... the platinum encourages your awareness to expand.... The spirals of light pour in all directions ... downwards ... upwards ... sideways ... forwards ... backwards.... Select a spiral on which to travel ... enter the vortex, knowing that you can move within it at your own pace.... Feel full of energy, vitality and power.... Be

aware of the soft strength within the vortex of your
choice.... Move from its wide part into its point ...
stretch out your hands ... touch the hard, cool and
comforting texture of granite.... Look down at your feet,
and see that you are standing on a six-pointed granite
star.... You are surrounded by an apricot cloud ... shot
through with silver light.... In your hand you hold a small
six-pointed platinum star ... the misty texture of apricot
around you is changing ... it is taking on the quality of
silk ... the granite star beneath you becomes the floor of a
silken tent.... From the top of the tent a bright, sharp,
silver beam strikes the centre of the platinum star held in
your hand ... the star refracts the light all around you and
into you.... Your whole being receives new vitality and
power.... Within your apricot silken tent you know that
you are part of a great universe beyond the imaginings of
the finite mind ... a universe which gains its vitality from
a divine place of regeneration ... an abundant place where
all things are possible.... The apricot, silken tent is a
revitalizing womb, which gives you healing, vitality and
power ... Stay here for as long as you wish and when you
are ready, gently return to the awareness of your
body.... Feel your feet in touch with the ground....
Draw a cloak of light with a hood around you ... become
fully aware of your normal, outer environment.

### 3.  Fragrances

Use the fragrances as suggested on pages 147. See pages
174 – 7 for further directions and suggestions for working
with fragrances.

### 4.  Colours

Locate the hara vortex in your auric field, strengthen the
connections to it from the sacral, solar plexus, liver and spleen
chakras, visualize its colours, but as well as breathing them
into the hara, feel them spiralling back into the connected

chakras and energizing them. Close down the petals, and picture in your mind the cross or star of light in a circle of light over your hara chakra to finish.

## 5.   The Prayer or Affirmation

Reflect or meditate on the words given on page 147.

## Chapter 14

# The Unconditional Love Centre

**Location**  Within and extending the usual heart chakra. (See fuller statement on page 74.)

**Key Words**  Wisdom, Unconditional Love, Self-Realization, Discrimination, Integrity

**Colours**  Rose, Amethyst, Pearlized Mauve

**Element**  Sea Water

**Quietening Fragrances**  Orchid, Camomile

**Stimulating Fragrances**  Geranium, Basil

**Crystals and Gemstones**  Amethyst, Sugilite (also called Luvulite), Lepidolite, Dolomite, Alexandrite

### Prayer or Affirmation

We open ourselves to the blessing of unconditional love. We accept that we are unconditionally loved. We ask that we may practise unconditional love without loss of integrity or wise discrimination. Help us to emerge from complacency.

## INTRODUCTORY COMMENTS

This is a 'centre' rather than a chakra. Its location is difficult to describe, but with patience and practice can be felt or realized as a deepening and extending of the heart chakra. Some guides have suggested that until recently the heart chakra we have experienced is the 'high heart' – slightly wrongly placed or developed in relationship to our physical bodies and over-limited in its scope. Opening the unconditional love centre rectifies this and opens new heart chakra potential.

## THE KEY WORDS

### Wisdom

This is one of the two archetypes for this centre. It awakens when the unconditional love centre is opened. It is the quality which comes when 'head and heart' are in harmony – when thinking is allied to warmth or compassion and emotion and feeling are tempered by thought.

### Unconditional Love

This is the second archetype – the one from which the centre takes its name. It is probably less difficult to give unconditional love than to believe that it is being given *to* us. The most difficult thing of all is to love ourselves. We are our own harshest critic or judge.

The prayer or affirmation asks that we may not lose 'wise discrimination' when practising unconditional love. We have to know where our own standards lie and to be clear about them. Unconditional love is not a blanket permission for 'anything goes'. Beyond reactive behaviour, the struggling spark or essence must always be given loving recognition. We need to be able to say to ourselves and others 'It *can* get better – *you* are not wrong. Your action or judgement may be questionable this time, but try again. I love you enough to help you do so.'

As an example here, it would mean nothing, in terms of unconditional love, to campaign or donate money for better conditions in prisons, unless you would also be prepared to meet prisoners as equal human beings, knowing that they may be carrying the human shadow for you, as much as for themselves. This quality is not born from superiority, distancing or over-detachment.

## Self-Realization

Self-realization is a phrase used by the psychologist, Maslow, to describe the moment or phase in life when we recognize our personal potential and decide to do something constructive about putting it into action. In time it leads to Self-Actualization, which is the conscious, effective use of all creative capacities and vision.

## Discrimination

The positive ability to be able to see for oneself what is good and true, without judgement of others who think or act differently. It is linked to integrity.

## Integrity

Dictionary definitions for this word are succinct and sufficient: wholeness, entirety, soundness, uprightness, honesty.

# THE COLOURS

Rose is a tender but full-bodied pink. Amethyst is the colour seen in those amethyst crystals which are rather pale in tone and have a tinge of grey within their hue. Pearlized Mauve is also light toned and slightly grey, with a pearly sheen. Lepidolite crystals shine with this colour.

Discarnate guides tell us that there is a whole range of

colour, as yet beyond our perception. When Gildas uses the word 'pearlized' he is endeavouring to describe a shade which is on the boundaries between that which we can see and that which is gradually coming into our vision.

## THE ELEMENT

Symbolically the sea usually is seen as feminine. (In French the word 'la mer' is almost the same as that for mother, i.e. la mère.) It also stands for the collective unconscious.

Sea-water is usually salty and tidal – a receptive, flowing yet powerful element whose hidden depths teem with life. Its rhythmic tides are governed by the moon. When the waters recede they draw things into their depths while high tides wash up flotsam, jetsam or hidden treasure. The flow and ebb causes stones on the beach to rub against each other, to change shape and reveal unexpected inner colour or texture.

Unconditional love is like the embrace of an all-accepting, though not all-protecting, parent who enables the rhythm of evolution to go on – until the true-self is revealed.

## THE FRAGRANCES

The unconditional love centre needs quietening in people who are over-anxious about their self-image and who feel unaccepted by others. It also helps those who become over-identified with or crushed by 'man's inhumanity to man'.

The stimulating fragrances are particularly helpful to people who feel that life is meaningless, shallow or nothing but a 'social round'.

## THE CRYSTALS AND GEMSTONES

Information on how to work with crystals and gemstones can be found on pages 174 – 7.

☆ *Amethyst* Stones chosen for the unconditional love centre should be pale or slightly greyish. They help the centre to awaken while also strengthening and protecting it.

☆ *Sugilite/Luvulite* is comparatively rare. It facilitates self-acceptance and encourages the development of feelings of unconditional love for self and others.

☆ *Lepidolite* is a form of mica. It aids forgiveness and release which are often necessary to the development of unconditional love.

☆ *Dolomite* strengthens the unconditional love centre and encourages the growth of integrity.

☆ *Alexandrite* helps in the cultivation of wise discrimination.

# MEDITATIONS AND SUGGESTIONS FOR DEVELOPING AND WORKING WITH YOUR UNCONDITIONAL LOVE CENTRE

## 1. Guided Visual Meditation for the Unconditional Love Centre

Let your body be comfortable, poised and symmetrical. . . . Be in touch with the rhythm of your breathing. . . . Gradually let this rhythm help you to bring the focus of your attention into your heart chakra . . . visualize each petal of the chakra opening rhythmically with each in-breath and out-breath. . . . Enter your own inner space and imagine that you are looking into a large, delicately scented, pink rose . . . notice the texture of the petals. . . . Each is tipped with a delicate touch of green . . . the centre of the flower is pure gold . . . The rose becomes large enough for you to enter into it . . . the gold in its centre becomes a golden gateway through which you can pass . . . into a garden beyond ... a rose garden ... full of mauve and pink roses.... It is formally laid out with grassed alleyways along which to walk and wooden seats under rose arbours.... Spend a little time exploring and perhaps sit for a while in one of the arbours.... Now you see a path which you have not previously noticed and you decide to follow it ... you leave the formal part of the garden and come to some rocks which shine with a pearly mauve light ... ahead of you is a rocky archway with an angel-like figure standing there ... as you come nearer to the archway and the being of light you know that you are welcome and that this guardian is not here to keep you out, but to welcome you and to protect you as you enter a specially sacred space.... You can now see an amethyst crystal temple ... as you come near the door opens and you go inside ... amethyst crystals are all around you ... giving a beautiful light and the atmosphere is warm and welcoming.... You find a comfortable place to sit and a sense of great peace and wellbeing envelops you ... you feel totally vulnerable and yet safe ... you know that you are fully accepted, fully seen and unconditionally loved.... Bask in this knowledge for a while.... When you are ready, retrace your steps ... out of the crystal temple, past the guardian at the archway, back through the formal rose garden to its golden gateway.... Go through the gateway ... and become aware again of your own breath in your heart chakra ... let the petals of this centre fold in and put a star or cross of light in a circle of light over it as a blessing.... Feel the contact of your feet with the ground and gradually ease back into your normal environment.

## 2.  Fragrances

Use the fragrances for this chakra, to activate, calm or balance it. See pages 33 – 5 for further directions and suggestions for working with fragrances.

## 3.  Colours

Find objects coloured with the unconditional love centre

shades shown on page 155. Glass or crystal is particularly good, since it gives the translucent quality of colour required. Study and absorb these colours, feel them affecting your heart centre and encouraging its deep inner part to awaken.

## 4. The Concept of Unconditional Love

Reflect on this. Which people in your life have offered you unconditional love and acceptance? Do you find this an easy quality to offer to others? Is it easy or difficult for you to accept and trust unconditional love? Seek a symbol or image for unconditional love.

## 5. The Prayer or Affirmation

Meditate or reflect on the words given on page 155.

# Chapter 15

# The Third Eye
# Chakra

**Location**  A vortex chakra, in the auric field, out from and slightly above the brow chakra.

**Key Words**  Beauty, Justice, Guardianship, Transformation

**Colours**  Silvery Blue, Indigo, Magenta

**Element**  Spiritual Fire

**Quietening Fragrances**  Carnation, Poppy

**Stimulating Fragrances** - Jasmine, Sage

**Crystals and Gemstones**  Optical Calcite, Ellestials, Herkimer Diamond, Fluorite Double Pyramids

### Prayer or Affirmation

We commit ourselves to vision. In this commitment we acknowledge that the vision of the past empowers the vision of the present and that the vision of the present enables the vision of the future. In service of that vision we ask the gifts of beauty and justice so that the structures of our security may be flexible and renewable. In making gold from the dross of life and experience, may we do so without despising the dross itself.

## INTRODUCTORY COMMENTS

The brow chakra is sometimes mistakenly called the 'third eye'. In reality these are two different centres and should not be confused. (See page 103 for brow chakra.) Like the hara chakra (page 147) the third eye is a vortex in the energy field. The energy structure on which it depends must be consciously strengthened before it can function properly. An exercise for accomplishing this is given on page 166.

The third eye is often spoken of in awed tones. People seeking a spiritual path will state 'learning to open the third eye' as a principal goal. There is confusion and glamour around what this exactly means. I have even been asked to perform an immediate third eye opening – presumably by some secret and magical intervention, psychic surgery or intercession!

The expectation seems to be compounded of wanting to be able to see past lives and future events; to shift levels of consciousness with ease; to astral travel; to diagnose and heal disease; to see auras and chakras; to see nature spirits and angels; and to have instant access to guidance. Many of these faculties are solar plexus based and psychic rather than spiritual in origin.

In fact, an open third eye means simply seeing life from a clear spiritual perspective; maintaining hope, faith and balance in a confusing and changing world; having a concept of oneself as a responsible spiritual guardian – and being able to develop the inner strength required for such a task; perceiving the inner quality of others without judgement and still loving them unconditionally. People who seriously attain these attitudes may well find that the gifts mentioned in the previous paragraph awaken naturally.

An open third eye is the reward for consistent application to spiritual development. It is a dangerous thing to possess without an accompanying psychological maturity and strong ego structure. To use the exercises given in this chapter is unwise, therefore, unless you have persevered with the rest of the journey through the chakras.

# THE KEY WORDS

## Beauty

This is the first archetype for this chakra. Standards of beauty are important in all civilizations. Experiments have proved that people most readily apply the adjectives 'beautiful' or 'harmonious' to architecture, illustrations and natural scenes which contain the 'golden mean'. (A proportion of 33⅓ to 66⅔, so that within an archway, for example, the top of the arch is approximately two-thirds as high as the wall in which it is set.) Natural form is based on proportions which have come to be called 'sacred geometry'. The third eye enables the true perception of beauty and helps to keep man-made structures in balance and harmony with nature.

## Justice

Justice is the second archetype for this centre. Every human community has to found a system of justice. Leaders who have a developed third eye establish wise boundaries and a legal system which is tempered with compassion.

## Guardianship

A quality of spirituality and maturity. When the third eye is functioning, harmonious living and wise guardianship of all resources becomes natural. Where this principle exists greed cannot.

## Transformation

Transformation is about 'change in form', with an inference that the final form reveals the potential held within the first. Thus a chrysalis transforms into a butterfly and an acorn becomes a mighty oak. The third eye chakra enables us to relate positively to the principle which Plato named 'entelechy' – the knowledge that the seed holds a blue-print of potential which will be actually and positively realized – the seed *will* 'become'.

# THE COLOURS

Silvery blue has a metallic quality. It is the colour seen in the chalcopyrites crystal Peacock Ore. Indigo has already been mentioned in connection with the brow chakra on page 107. Magenta is a reddish violet. Although violet is usually given as the colour having the highest vibrational rate within the known spectrum, some shades of magenta vibrate even faster. It may therefore be the first colour of a higher octave gradually revealing itself to our perception.

These are the colours which the third eye causes to flow into the auric field. Visualizing them and feeding them into the third eye will nourish and awaken it.

# THE ELEMENT

Spiritual fire is quite different from elemental fire. It inspires that quality of being which has idealism and zest within it.

In inner reality spiritual fire is the flame which purifies and cleanses without consuming.

# THE FRAGRANCES

The quietening fragrances should be used by people who are over-anxious about acquiring special gifts or where there has been an accelerated development of psychic faculties.

The stimulating oils should be used with discretion and alongside a chakra development programme which includes attention to the whole system.

A balancing fragrance can be made by mixing all four perfumes given on page 162.

## THE CRYSTALS AND GEMSTONES

Information on how to work with crystals and gemstones can be found on pages 174 – 7.

☆ *Optical Calcite* is a clear version of calcite, with a rhomboid form. It breaks light into the spectrum of colour and is therefore full of rainbows. True to its name, it aids clear sight and vision of a spiritual nature.

☆ *Ellestials* are among the more recent crystal discoveries. They have a similar appearance to smoky quartz but their form is square and flat. They form close clusters and often have water trapped within them. They are crystals which inspire and encourage us to reach out for our highest potential.

☆ *Herkimer Diamond* is a member of the quartz family. They are diamond shaped crystals, usually quite small and clear as though having been polished and faceted. They are only mined in Herkimer County, New York State and grow in liquid solution. They enhance all spiritual qualities, give vitality and encourage joy.

☆ *Fluorite Double Pyramids* are also diamond shaped. They aid the development of spiritual awareness and help to transform spiritual ideas into material reality. They come in different shades, mainly white, purple, mauve and green. The white or purple are most suitable for the third eye.

## MEDITATIONS AND SUGGESTIONS FOR DEVELOPING AND WORKING WITH YOUR THIRD EYE CHAKRA

### 1.   Building the Subtle Structure
Make sure that you will be undisturbed and then let your body be comfortable, poised and symmetrically

arranged.... Be in touch with the rhythm of your breathing.... Try to sense your aura as an energy that surrounds you just beyond the flesh of your physical body.... Feel the area where your brow chakra emerges into this field ... focus your attention a little beyond it and above it and seek a spot of more intense energy .... (If you are a healer or have a naturally developed third eye you may already be able to sense a moving vortex of energy.) Sense the colours of silvery blue ... indigo ... and magenta. Now visualize a line of energy going from this area of your auric field into your brow chakra and through from there to connect with the pineal gland (see page 108) ... breathe along this line, visualizing it full of light, strong and clear.... Imagine another line of energy running from the third eye position up to the crown chakra ... breathe strength into it.... Another energy line goes through the petals of the alter major and into its stem, while a fourth travels to the throat chakra.... Visualize each in turn and work to strengthen them.... Return your attention to the third eye itself and see whether the vortex is clearer, stronger or has more movement in it.... Spend not longer than 15 minutes per day with this exercise. When you have finished feel your feet in contact with the ground and focus back into your outer world.... Imagine a cloak of white light, with a hood, drawn around you.

## 2. Guided Visual Meditation for the Third Eye Chakra

Making sure that you will be undisturbed let your body be comfortable, poised and symmetrically arranged.... Be in touch with the rhythm of your breathing and let this rhythm help you to focus your attention into the area of your third eye chakra ... a vortex in your auric field, slightly above the brow chakra petals.... Be aware of the cords of light which connect this vortex with the brow, pineal, crown, alter major and throat chakras.... Feel the third eye vortex moving more strongly as you explore and strengthen its connecting cords and prepare for an inner journey. . . . Imagine yourself entering the third eye vortex . . . being drawn into its centre, where you are surrounded by the colours of silvery blue . . . indigo and magenta. . . . The centre of the vortex is like a well of bright indigo light. . . . You are drawn towards it . . . and experience it like an eye. . . . You look through the eye into a bright world beyond . . . and then you step through . . . the light is very clear and you can see a long way into a beautiful landscape. . . . As you walk in this special light you find yourself reflecting on the qualities of beauty, justice, guardianship and transformation. . . . You come to a meadow . . . and, looking around, see wondrous flowers . . . they are unlike any you have ever seen or imagined before . . . some shine with silvery blue, others are indigo, magenta and gold. . . . You pick a flower of each colour . . . within the silvery blue flower lies a symbol for beauty . . . within the indigo flower a symbol for justice . . . within the magenta a symbol for guardianship and within the golden flower a symbol for transformation. . . . You can carry these symbols anywhere you wish, in your chakras or body. . . . Decide where you will place them . . . and then carry them as a sign of your commitment to fresh vision and spiritual awareness. . . . As you place the last symbol within, you know that it is time to return. . . . You are drawn back through the pupil of the indigo eye . . . into the vortex . . . into your physical body . . . back to the awareness of your breath and to full consciousness of your everyday surroundings. . . . Put a cloak of white light, with a hood right around you, feel your feet on the ground, return fully to the outer world.

## 3.   Fragrances

Use the fragrances for this chakra as suggested on page 162. See pages 35 – 5 for directions and suggestions for the use of fragrances with the chakras.

## 4.   The Prayer or Affirmation

Meditate and reflect on the words given on page 162.

# Chapter 16
# Answers to Common Questions

**How do you sense a chakra?**

The ability to do this grows quite quickly with practice and perseverance. Before you begin to sense a particular chakra familiarize yourself with the central column exercises on pages 7 – 9.

Concentrate on one chakra at a time, read the location note at the beginning of its chapter and study the diagram on page 5. Relax, and focus your attention on the relevant part of your body. Imagine invisible, flower-like petals projecting into your energy field. Know that the chakra energy interpenetrates with your physical body and feeds into the central column. It then moves into the stem which is a tube-like protuberance into the energy field at the back. There is directional flow from the petals to the stem and out through it. (Reversed only in the case of the alter major chakra.)

Rub your hands together and hold them gently over the petals of the chakra which you wish to sense. Use your breath to help you bring your attention into the appropriate area. Think about the following words: alive; asleep; awake; bright; closed; cold; flexible; numb; open; over-active; pale; pulsating; tender; tight; tingling; turning; under-active; warm.

Associate one or more of these words, or a feeling quality suggested by them to the chakra with which you are working. Write down your impressions.

Take a selection of crayons. Check the energies in your chakra again and intuitively draw them in colour. Choosing the crayons with your left hand will activate your intuition more strongly. (This applies whether you are normally left-handed or not.) After a while, you will realize that you are sensing the energies and colours in your chakras quite easily. You will become sensitive to changes in them and more confident with the colour 'feeding' exercises first described on page 39. If you have a friend or partner interested in working with you, practise sensing each other's chakras. Discussing your findings will give you a firmer frame of reference. Try to be aware of your first and immediate impressions and to resist interpreting or analysing your findings too soon.

**I am suspicious of my own findings. How can I be sure that I am not inventing or imagining it all?**

Many people feel uneasy about the parts their mind or imagination play in sensing and contacting the subtle realms. We are conditioned to believe that only outer, tangible things are genuine. We are taught to make distinctions between imaginary and real. It is not easy to make the shift into recognizing that each different area of the psyche has a reality of its own.

When you are exploring subtle areas and something comes 'to mind', it is more likely to be true than untrue. Why should this particular thought come, at this particular time, out of all the permutations that would have been possible? Most likely because it is pertinent to the immediate situation.

Imagination is creative and playful, but when you are in touch with inner reality, whether you have 'imagined' it into being or not, the things which are true or enduring are not subject to facile change. That which persists should be trusted.

## How can I develop my ability to visualize?

Check whether you are blocking your ability to visualize by any of the considerations commented on in response to the previous question.

We are all much more visual in our approach to life than may be generally recognized. If you habitually buy one particular brand of washing powder, it is unlikely that you only recognize it on the supermarket shelf by carefully reading its name on the packet. You carry an image of what you expect it to look like and using this, can quickly pick out your brand from the others. This is a form of visualization, only confused when the manufacturer changes the packaging – particularly the colours.

Visualization is a combination of imagination and inner sensing. Inner vision does not follow the same rules as outer sight. Thinking about something, or having sensations or vague intimations are all part of the process. Do not be too ready to condemn yourself as a non-visualizer. Find and respect the way in which you *do* get inner knowledge. A little self-appreciation goes a long way in cultivating the refined faculties.

Right brain enthusiasts, in reaction to society's over-emphasis on intellect and logic, have tended to imply that 'thinking' is a dirty word. To be in balance, we need an easy access to all our faculties. Valuing your strong areas will help you find creative ways of developing the weaker ones. (See *Glossary* for further information on the right and left brain.)

If visualization is not easy, one of your other senses may help you in the inner realms. Can you first smell, touch, hear or taste and thus encourage the image to follow? Try spontaneously to draw or write without feeling that you have to reach some esoteric altered state of consciousness in order to get results.

## Can you say more about the chakra polarities?

Like an electrical circuit, chakras have a positive and negative polarity. It could also be said that they have an 'earth' terminal where they feed into the central column. All except the alter major, third eye, unconditional love centre and hara have their positive polarity in the petals and negative in the stem. The alter major has reversed polarity while the other three chakras mentioned are of a completely different form. The negative polarity of the crown and the root chakras is inside the central column at either end, as are their stems.

The flow in a chakra is from positive polarity to negative – in through the petals and out through the stem, always excepting the alter major, where the energy goes in through the stem and out through the petals. A healthy directional flow is essential to a healthy chakra.

Most healers find that they have a positive polarity flow from their right hands and a negative polarity flow from their left. This makes the right hand directional and the left hand receptive. When balancing and healing chakras they often, therefore, hold the right hand over the petals and the left over the stem, channelling light and energy in to the positive polarity and drawing out anything which needs to be given off with the left hand at the stem. (Always reversed for the alter major. Positive and negative polarities in the hands when used for healing does not depend on right or left handedness.)

**I should like to know more about the meaning of colours.**

In terms of inner work, understanding the chakras and their keywords give a fuller insight into the meaning of colour. Each chakra is responsible for producing a particular colour, which then feeds our energetic field. Without a full colour spectrum, we are not completely healthy. Colours which are too intense often indicate emotional upset or imbalance. Weak or pale colours may result from exhaustion or physical illness. Balancing the colours through visualization or receiving healing will help the recuperative process.

As well as producing a specific colour each chakra also has its own intrinsic spectrum. Any colour may appear in any or every chakra. The distribution of colours will thus give further information about the way we are, or our potential.

To summarize briefly, red is the root chakra colour and denotes the ability to relate to incarnation. 'Red energy' is often seen as sexual, but sensual is more accurate. Because of its intensity, red should be taken in small doses. For healing and visualization it is usually modified to a deep-toned pinky red.

If red is seen in other chakras, it will mean that the energy of that chakra is easily directed into the physical world and the concerns of incarnation. Someone with red in their heart chakra, for instance, is likely to be compassionate to those who are materially deprived.

Orange is produced by the sacral chakra and signifies vitality, creativity, sexuality and power. Seen in another chakra it will signify that these qualities are enhancing, or blending with its own. Successful athletes usually have orange in their solar plexus and/or throat chakras.

The solar plexus gives us yellow, which is a colour of confidence, focus and mental ability. Yellow in the heart chakra can indicate someone who is detached from their feelings, but often the victim of their emotions. In the throat chakra it will show the ability to gather factual information and to communicate it clearly. Mathematicians usually have yellow at the throat.

Green is the colour of the heart and stands for compassion, wisdom, detachment and tenderness. In the sacral and/or throat chakras it would denote the poet, artist, visionary or writer with a message for society. Teachers and social workers often have green at the solar plexus.

Blue, given out by the throat, is the colour of communication, expression, purpose and healing. The throat has a natural link to the sacral chakra, and blue there would suggest the healer or priest, as might indigo.

Indigo is produced by the brow. It is the colour of the spirit and of high aspiration. Appearing in other centres it will require the energy of that chakra to be dedicated to higher service. Monks and nuns drawn to contemplative orders may have a lot of indigo in the root, sacral and solar plexus chakras. People who find it difficult to reconcile spirituality and sexuality will tend to have indigo in their sacral chakras.

Violet and gold, produced by the crown chakra, are soul colours. Seen in other chakras they will imply that the individual is aware of, or needs to awaken to a sense of destiny. Great leaders and true rulers have these colours at the throat, solar plexus and heart.

Obviously colour is a big subject, but this information added to that in each chakra chapter should help you, as your sensitivity develops, to read your chakras more accurately.

## Can you say more about how to use the crystals?

The descriptions of the crystals in each chakra chapter show which qualities the different types will develop, encourage, or enhance.

Crystals are readily available from many different shops, suppliers or market stalls. Use the crystal sections in each chapter to help you to decide which varieties of stones you would like to acquire. When you have found a source, rely on your intuition to tell you which, of a particular variety, is the right crystal for you.

Spend some time getting to know your crystal. Look at it carefully, handle it, admire it. When you are ready to prepare it for serious work, wait until three days before the full moon, and put it into water containing a little sea salt. Do not do this with crystals mounted as jewellery, with synthetic crystals, or with those which feel soft or flaky – such as lepidolite. These can be frequently rinsed in running water during this period, or placed on a large, previously cleansed, amethyst cluster.

On the night of the full moon dry the crystal on silk or soft cotton and put it in the garden or on the windowsill. Don't worry if the full moon is behind cloud, the crystal will absorb what it needs. After this, it should be 'charged' by twelve hours of sunlight. (Behind glass is fine, but the light should shine as directly as possible on to the crystal which should be turned regularly.) This charging can be done intermittently until twelve hours' worth of sun has been absorbed.

In a simple ceremony dedicate the crystal to its purpose. Light a candle, hold the stone for a while in your cupped hands, and then ask it to help in your development or healing.

When the crystal is cleansed and dedicated, it does not matter whether you place it in one of your rooms, wear it in a special bag around your neck, or put it by your bed or under your pillow. You can direct its energies more specifically, when you want to.

As well as asking your crystals to enhance your dreams and meditations or to help you focus on developing a specific quality, they can be used for healing, charging, cleansing and developing your chakras.

Some crystals most often come in a piece without individual crystals growing out of them – rose quartz, malachite, carnelian, calcite and jasper are examples. Unless they have been cut or polished into a wand they have no defined polarities. Their energy is receptive, calming, feminine and yin. They are often referred to as crystals of massive form.

Other crystals have one end which is faceted and pointed and the other more rounded or less defined – clear quartz, amethyst, citrine, and celestite come most often in this form, either singly or as clusters. In these cases the pointed end is positive in polarity, directive, energizing, masculine and yang, while the other is negative in polarity, receptive, calming, feminine and yin. These crystals, having a defined, faceted end are often called 'terminated crystals'.

Massive form crystals can be used for general healing and calming of the chakras, as well as to aid the development of the specific chakra qualities with which the crystal may be linked. Just hold the stone on or over the chakra petals, relax, reflect and meditate on the help you wish the crystal to focus for you. Do not spend longer than five minutes per chakra.

The terminated crystals, either singly or in clusters may be used to charge a chakra with energy. Clear quartz are particularly good for this as they are so versatile in their use. If you feel that a chakra is depleted or you know that you are going to need a particular chakra to be more vital than usual to cope with a specific situation – for example, the solar plexus to help you cope with some stress or an examination – hold the directive, faceted end over the chakra petals for two or three minutes while you concentrate on breathing deeply into the chakra. To start with, only hold the directive point of a crystal directly over a chakra for two to three minutes at a time. They are dynamic and you need to assess their effect on you carefully.

The receptive end of a single terminated crystal or crystal cluster can be used to help a chakra to close in after meditation or guided visualization, by holding it over the chakra petals while you are visualizing the cross or star in the circle of light.

The flow in a chakra, from petals to stem is aided by directing the point of a single terminated crystal at the chakra petals while you breathe in and then imagine the out-breath going out through the stem. This helps the chakra to cleanse and energize itself. Some chakras, particularly the sacral and solar plexus, benefit from having the petals cleansed by making a gentle scooping or spooning movement over the petals with the terminated end of a single crystal or crystal cluster.

Terminated crystal can also be used to 'comb' your aura. It may be easier to get someone else to do this for you. Starting just above the head, with the faceted end towards the aura, make long sweeps down to the feet, always travelling in a downward direction. (Hold the crystal well away from the energy field as you bring it up to commence the next sweep.) This can be done with the recipient sitting on a stool or dining chair or lying down. If lying down it is necessary to turn over to do the back, as the whole auric field should be thoroughly combed. Do at least ten long combing strokes. This technique is helpful before sleep, if you have been involved in emotionally stressful situations, or at the end of a healing session.

There is only space here to mention the most common crystal forms, but there are several good crystal books available if you want to extend your knowledge. These are mentioned in the Bibliography.

Remember to wash working crystals frequently under running water. When they are at rest they like to lie on a piece of silk, or cotton velvet.

### Does massage help the chakras? Can you say something about the different forms of massage?

Where the need for root chakra work is indicated there is usually a need to be more in touch with the body. For this purpose full Swedish body massage is recommended. This is a firm massage which tones muscles and encourages the release of toxins. For the sacral chakra lymphatic drainage massage may be useful.

Aromatherapy can apply to the recommendation of specific oils to put in the bath or environment or it may be combined with Swedish massage, lymphatic drainage, reflexology, intuitive massage, or etheric massage.

Reflexologists work on the feet. All the chakras and all the organs of the body have corresponding energy points in the feet. The parts of the foot which are tender or give pain when pressed or massaged will enable a reflexologist to diagnose trouble spots in the body. Massaging or applying pressure to these points will stimulate the vital systems and promote healing.

Intuitive masseurs tune in to their client's needs and massage the body with firm or light pressure accordingly.

A certain amount of etheric massage is used by most healers. The aura combing exercise with a crystal given on page 176 is a form of etheric massage. Stroking the body with a very light touch, combined with holding the hands still over chakra points or vital organs strengthens the etheric layer and helps to provide the balance and vitality necessary to full bodily healing.

Combing, scooping and stroking the chakra areas is beneficial, either with light touch on the body or mainly concentrating on the auric field. The alter major positive polarity point benefits from gentle, circular massage and stroking with the finger tips. Other chakras should not be massaged over the petals with circular movements and crystals or pendulums should not be swung directly above them. They have their own rhythm, pulsation and movement and circular motion over them tends to interfere with this rather than enhance it.

**Could you say more about chakra pairs and the extent to which it is wise to work with one chakra alone?**

Always keep in mind that the chakras form a team. If one member in the team is out of balance then individual work must be done with that member, but to work exclusively with one chakra over too long a period could create fresh team imbalances. This hazard can be avoided by always working with the heart or root chakra as well as the imbalanced chakra, or by working with one or other of its natural pairs. Thus: the root pairs with the heart and the crown; the sacral with the throat; the solar plexus with the brow and the crown; the alter major with the root, crown or sacral; the base with the root; the hara with the sacral; the unconditional love centre with the heart; and the third eye with the brow. It will be seen that the main chakra pairs are between complementary colours: root/red with heart/green; sacral/orange with throat/blue; solar plexus/yellow with brow/indigo and crown/violet.

Each chakra may also be paired with the one directly below or above itself. This is a particularly useful way of working when dealing with emotional issues.

# Chapter 17

# A Reflection on Some of the Chakra Energies of Our Time

As the human body has chakras, so does the body of the earth. Many suggestions have been offered as to where the main planetary chakras lie. In truth there are so many inter-linking energy systems around the globe that any mapping of its chakra system is fraught with difficulty. Each country, each area, even each town or village has its own complete chakra system. Working with your own chakras gives you a basic idea of the feel and function of the major centres. It can then be fun and instructive to try to sense local energies.

The making of pilgrimages helps to keep life force flowing between one chakra point and another. Today there is a revival of this act of service. One chakra system which seems relatively clear and marked is that which runs from the South of France to the North of Scotland. It is currently attracting many conscious and unconscious pilgrims. There is a strong root chakra area which begins at Les Saintes Maries de la Mer in the Camargue. It is here that Mary the Mother of Christ, Mary the mother of St John the Divine and Mary Magdalene are said to have arrived by boat after the crucifixion of Jesus. They were accompanied by St John the Divine and a dark-skinned servant called Sarah who has a shrine in the crypt of the church at Les Saintes Maries. She is revered by most true gypsies, who annually converge in this swampy area to worship at 'their' shrine.

The sacral chakra begins at the level of Clermont Ferrand and the solar plexus at Chartres. The Channel between France and England is symbolic of the lack of communication which often exists between the lower chakras and the heart. London is the centre of the heart chakra, the throat is in Yorkshire, with Durham Cathedral a strong centre for throat chakra energy. The alter major chakra takes in Northumberland, the brow has Edinburgh as its centre and the crown is in the North of Scotland, including the holy Isle of Iona.

Apart from reflecting on where the chakras are in the body of the earth it is interesting to see the reflection of their energies and developmental stages in human nature – the body of humanity.

A 'chakra case history' of humanity in 1993 must first point out an over-active solar plexus. The speed of change makes each organisation, race or country uncertain of its identity. We could be said to be in an identity crisis. In Eastern Europe there is a fight for territory – this may well be one of the major solar plexus chakra areas of the earth.

At such times the solar plexus chakra is not sufficiently linked to the brow or the crown. The church has traditionally been the vehicle for these higher energies, but it is no longer attracting enough people or offering solutions or solace in our difficulties. The balance of power lies with the lower, rather than the higher, will. We need a major spiritual awakening to bring about a cleansing of the brow and crown chakras and a realignment of them with the solar plexus.

The solar plexus is connected with digestion. Certain sectors of humanity have become motivated by greed. The digestive system has been thrown into chronic dis-array – so much so that the body of humanity is exhibiting serious indications of dis-ease.

The plight of the third world is one of the most acute

symptoms. There are enough resources on the planet to feed, clothe and shelter all who inhabit her but the distribution is at fault. Vital organs are being affected. Lessons about wholesome nurturing, from the root chakra and the wise use of power, from the sacral, have not been assimilated.

There must be care that the system does not go into heart attack or total stress breakdown. The opening of the unconditional love centre offers the possibility of strengthening and healing humanity's heart.

The throat chakra is strong. Our communication systems are sophisticated and the plight of vital organs or members can be registered. If the heart is enabled to respond to the information voiced by the throat, seeds of hope may be planted and allowed to germinate.

The new chakras also offer channels for healing. The base puts us more in touch with the privilege of being on the earth as part of the brotherhood/sisterhood of humanity. The hara and third eye give us new energy resources and perspectives. The third eye will also help to revitalise the brow and crown chakras. The alter major chakra will sharpen our instincts and enable a unified response to their distress signals.

That which begins in the individual permeates through to the whole. One of the subtly powerful contributions we can make to the realignment of humanity, is to work with our chakra systems and so make our contribution to more vital, healthy and spiritually harmonious living within the body of humanity.

# Glossary

**Angelic Beings** These are direct reflections of Divine Consciousness. They are intermediaries and guardians helping the Divine plan to manifest on earth. Their hierarchy includes Guardian Angels, Archangels, Cherubim and Seraphim.

The elemental/devic/angelic hierarchy or lifestream may be seen as moving from the divine consciousness towards earth, while the human stream of consciousness which includes discarnate guides, may be seen to be moving towards reunification with the Divine. Thus the elemental/devic/angelic hierarchy is separate from humanity. Discarnates are not angels and angels will not take on human form or consciousness. Our Guardian Angels are thus different from our guides or discarnate mentors.

**Anima/Animus** These are Jungian terms. (From C. G. Jung the psychologist.) An important part of personality integration, whatever our gender, is to come to terms with both the masculine and feminine principles. These are present in each one of us. The inner feminine in a man is called the 'Anima' and the inner masculine in a woman, the 'Animus'.

**Akasha** This is usually considered to be a fifth element. There is a progression from the tangible earth, water, fire and air, to the intangible akasha or ether. It is like a collective subtle body for humanity, holding the imprint of everything each individual, group, family or race has ever known, done or is in the process of knowing and doing. It is also thought to have a relationship to the origin of sound and colour. Akasha is approximately the same as that which Jung described as the 'collective unconscious'.

**Archetypes** By dictionary definition these are 'primordial images inherited by all'. Each human society is affected by forces such as peace, war, beauty, justice, wisdom, healing, death, birth, love, power. The essence of these defies definition and we need images, myths, symbols and personifications to help us in understanding the depth and breadth of them. Tarot cards, which have ancient origins, have twenty-two personified or symbolized archetypes in the major arcana. These cover all aspects of human experience.

**Astral plane/body/travel** The astral plane is the layer which comes after the etheric (see page 67). It is a complex area of consciousness having many levels. Much, though not all, dream experience takes place on the astral plane. In an altered state of consciousness it is possible to contact the astral layer. There is an immediate difference of feeling quality. A client described the change thus: 'Whereas at one point I knew my imagery to be a very real part of my inner world, I was the sole creator. The figures I met were parts of my present personality. When the change came I knew that not only was my guide appearing to me, but I was appearing to him.'

The higher layers of the astral plane contain healing temples and ethereal landscapes which we certainly visit after death and where we may work in the after-death state.

If we die with a rather rigid thought form about the after-death state, such as the expectation that we shall live happily with a previously deceased loved one in a cottage in the country with roses around the door, we go for a while to the middle astral zone and experience that idyll until we are ready to release it and move on. Those who speak through mediums from the after-death state in the same personality form as they had in life, need to come to the middle astral zone in order to do so. Higher guides and teachers usually speak from the feeling or mental planes (see pages 81 and 95).

Many people express the desire for 'astral travel', not realizing that they may already be travelling to the astral plane in their dreams. They usually mean that they want to be able to enter their astral body in order to travel to other places on the material plane. We may be prevented from doing this simply because such travel can be an intrusion on the privacy of others – but the ability can be developed and a specialist teacher should be consulted. When near-death experiences are described there is often mention of 'floating' above the physical body, looking down on it, knowing what is being done to help it and who is present, but feeling detachment and no pain. At such times the whole consciousness has entered the astral body but is still linked to the physical body.

The lower astral planes are full of thought forms and entities. These may be encountered in nightmares, on bad drug trips, when inebriated or during some types of psychotic episode. When chakra energies are being wisely explored and managed there is no danger of being caught up in these unpleasant areas during meditation and visualization – but if you have any fears around this possibility speak to a spiritual counsellor or meditation teacher.

**Aura** An energy field, which interpenetrates with and radiates out beyond the physical body. It has various frequencies vibrating within it, which are called subtle bodies. Clairvoyantly seen, the aura is full of light, colour and shade. The trained healer or seer sees, within the aura, indications as to the spiritual, mental, physical and emotional state of the individual. Much of the auric colour and energy comes from the chakras.

**Devic Beings** These may sometimes be confused with angels. A deva is a good, shining spirit and often very tall. Their concern is with trees, rocks, plants, animals, and the four elements. They are guardians who work to maintain balance in these realms and in the interaction of humanity with the natural kingdoms.

**Ego** The present conscious personality; what we mean when we say 'I'.

**Elementals** Tiny energy beings generally associated with plants, trees, the natural environment and the elements. They appear to those who 'see' as points of light or colour or in traditional fairy form as the nereids, sylphs, gnomes, elves, undines etc of fairy tales.

Since the four elements interact in our physical bodies and largely determine our health patterns, elementals are within and around us. Healing energy activates and encourages them to help us to health and harmony.

Elementals are the lowest manifestation in a hierarchy of a different consciousness stream from the human. Above them are Devic Beings and Angels.

**Inner Child** Within each one of us there is a child self, which has many aspects. If our actual childhood has been traumatic then the child self will be confused and needy and will have to be reclaimed and healed. When this work is successful the spirit of the inner child which maintains truthfulness, naturalness, spontaneity and creativity can be released – we can know innocence and wisdom at one and the same time and rediscover our true selves.

**Karma** The spiritual law of cause and effect (which defies 'nutshell' definition). 'As you sow, so shall you reap', gives a basic but over-simplified idea. Belief in karma goes alongside belief in reincarnation and personal, progressive evolution. The tendency is to see karma as being something troublesome or heavy which needs to be overcome during a specific lifetime – but giftedness or innate wisdom are positive karmic attributes.

**Kirlian Photography** This is an electrical form of photography, discovered in Russia. It enables the energy field of humans, animals, plants, minerals, food etc to be registered and printed similarly to conventional photography. Auric or energy-field colours also show in a Kirlian photograph. Trained observers or interpreters can make diagnoses as to physical, mental and emotional health, from the prints.

**Psyche** Analytic and transpersonal psychologies have shown how complex the human personality is. The psyche refers to the total being, with all its drives, needs, conflicts, disease, health, gifts and potential.

**Right Brain/Left Brain** The most active part of the brain is divided into two hemispheres. The left hemisphere controls the right side of the body and vice versa. The left brain governs cognitive learning – language, facts, figures and abstract thought. The right brain governs our more imaginative functions – art, symbolism, dreams, intuition and the autonomous systems of our bodies. Right brain imagery is thus a valuable tool in self-healing.

The tendency in the Western world is to place more value on left brain functions. The ideal is to have both sides of the brain coordinated, as well as being able to call on the advantages of each at will.

**Shadow** The part of the 'I' which we do not admit into full consciousness. That which is unconscious, undefined, formless, dark, shadowy and without concept. The unknown.

**Subtle Bodies** Beyond the physical body, forming the auric field, are subtle bodies or energy layers, each having a different frequency or vibration. Through these bodies links with the wider being are maintained and remembered.

At death the subtle bodies live on and 'clothe' the spirit as it passes to the other side.

The total number of subtle bodies accepted by most sources is six. (Seven bodies altogether, including the physical.) Terminology for these varies. In this book, moving outwards from the physical, they are called: the etheric body; the astral body; the feeling body; the lower mental body; the higher mental body; and the ketheric, soul or causal body. There is a subdivision of the causal body linked to the alter major chakra and called the lower causal body.

**Transpersonal Psychology** The dictionary meaning of the word psychology is 'the study of human behaviour'. At a scientific level this means the actual study of human reflexes, learning mechanisms, perception, needs, drives, etc. There are a number of schools of 'behavioural psychology' which arise from such study.

Transpersonal psychology addresses the spiritual needs and aspirations of human beings as well as the behavioural. It concentrates on the importance of finding a meaning in life and of being creative and fulfilled in living and relating.

**Yin and Yang** These are Chinese words for the basic but opposite aspects of creation. Yin is receptive, feminine and dark. Yang is active, masculine and light. In the traditional yin/yang symbol one black and one white fish-like shape nestle together to form a perfect circle. The eye of the black shape is white and of the white shape black, showing that the seed of each is contained in the other.

# Bibliography

Anodea, Judith, *Wheels of Life*, Distributor: W. Foulsham
Bailey, Alice, *Discipleship in the New Age*, The Lucius Trust
Barnard, Christian, *The Body Machine*, Hamlyn
Burckhardt, Titus, *Alchemy*, Element Books
Cooper, J. C., *The Aquarian Dictionary of Festivals*, Aquarian
  and *An Illustrated Encyclopedia of Traditional Symbols*, Thames
  and Hudson
Claremont di Castiliego, Catherina, *Knowing Woman*,
  Shambhala Publications
Holbeche, Soozi, *The Power of Gems and Crystals* and *The Power
  of Your Dreams*, Piatkus Books
Raphaell, Katharina, *Crystal Enlightenment* and *Crystal
  Healing*, Aurora Press
White, Ruth, *A Question of Guidance*, C. W. Daniel Co. Ltd.
White, Ruth and Swainson, Mary, *Gildas Communicates*,
  C. W. Daniel Co. Ltd.

# Index

**Ruth White** leads many workshops on a variety of subjects in London, other areas of Britain and in several European countries. She also runs an 18-month training course for healers, a one-year leadership course and channelling courses, all based in London. Information is available from:

Dragon's Den
3 Manor Farm Lane
Tidmarsh
Nr. Reading
Berkshire RG8 8EY

Meditative tapes for each chakra featuring meditations spoken by Ruth and sounds for the chakras made by Susannah Tyrell are available from:

Mike Finesilver
Pathway Studio
2a Grosvenor Avenue
London N5 2NR

Further details and a price list will be sent on request.

# PIATKUS BOOKS

If you are interested in the Mind, Body and Spirit area, you may like to read other titles published by Piatkus.

PIATKUS